EUROHIP

Karsten E. Dreinhöfer • Paul Dieppe
Klaus-Peter Günther • Wolfhart Puhl

Editors

EUROHIP

Health Technology Assessment of Hip Arthroplasty in Europe

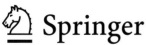

Editors

Karsten E. Dreinhöfer
Department of Orthopaedics
University of Ulm
Oberer Eselsberg 45
89081 Ulm
Germany
karsten.dreinhoefer@uni-ulm.de
and
MEDICAL PARK Berlin Humboldtmühle
Department of Orthopaedics,
Traumatology and Sports Medicine
An der Mühle 2-9
13507 Berlin
Germany
k.dreinhoefer@medicalpark.de

Klaus-Peter Günther
Department of Orthopaedics
UniversitätsklinikumCarl Gustav Carus
Fetscherstr. 74
01307 Dresden
Germany
klaus-peter.guenther@uniklinikum-dresden.de

Paul Dieppe
University of Bristol
Department of Social Medicine
Canynge Hall
Whiteladies Road
Bristol BS8 2PR
United Kingdom
and
Peninsula College of Medicine
and Dentistry
University of Plymouth Campus
Drake Circus
Plymouth, PL4 8AA
United Kingdom
paul.dieppe@pms.ac.uk

Wolfhart Puhl
University of Ulm
Oberer Eselsberg
89081 Ulm
Germany
and
Department of Special
Orthopedic Surgery
Klinik Oberstdorf
Trettachstr. 16
87561 Oberstdorf
Germany
wolfhart.puhl@efort.org

ISBN: 978-3-540-74133-6   e-ISBN: 978-3-540-74137-4
DOI: 10.1007/978-3-540-74137-4
Springer Dordrecht Heidelberg London New York

Library of Congress Control Number: 2009921796

Cover design: F. Steinen-Broo, eStudio Calamar, Spain

Printed on acid-free paper

Springer is part of Springer Science+Business Media (www.springer.com)

Projects have the greatest chance of success if the underlying question carries weight and is cogently put.

Successful projects get off to the best start in the most favourable circumstances, for example when a clearly targeted question is brought together with vision and drive.

The 'EUROHIP' project was initiated in just such propitious conditions on 28 October 1997 when Reinhard Mohn and Wolfhart Puhl sat opposite each other to talk about the indication for surgery in coxarthritis. Reinhard Mohn had to accept that there were indeed different ways of looking at the indication.

Following a frank question and answer session, he found himself able to support Puhl's basic argument. However, on account of his analytical approach and his constant desire to find answers to open questions, and to resolve any unsolved problems, he remained dissatisfied with the overall situation.

His proposal, therefore, was to collect comparative data from all over Europe as a means of finding a substantiated solution which was basically acceptable to all parties.

All those working on the "Eurohip" project and all patients who stand to benefit from this work are grateful.

Following its introduction to routine medical care in the 1960s, total hip joint replacement has become one of the most valuable interventions available for chronic pain and disability. It has been shown to be both effective and cost-effective, and in all developed countries of the world demand and provision have both risen steadily over the last three decades. But in spite of the clear success of total hip replacement, practice variations remain huge, and many scientific questions about its provision are still to be answered.

Most developed countries are struggling to finance first class health care for everyone in their community, leading to renewed emphasis on appropriate and equitable provision of health care, and putting interventions that are both high in volume and expense under the microscope. Purchasers and managers of health care provision in Europe are now demanding answers to some of the unanswered questions about hip replacement.

The Eurohip project has been set up to try to answer some of these questions. With the help of funding from the Bertelsmann Foundation and Centrepulse Orthopaedic Ltd. (Sulzer Medical Ltd.) we were able to create a collaboration involving 22 orthopaedic centres from 12 different European countries. This collaboration is undertaking several different investigations into hip replacement, to address indications, practice variations, costs and outcomes. It is affiliated with the 'Bone and Joint Decade'.

We would like to acknowledge the hard work that Karsten Dreinhöfer has put into the Eurohip project. Without his help, the projects being undertaken, in addition to the publication of this book, would not have been possible.

Wilfred von Eiff
Paul Dieppe
Wolfhart Puhl
Principal Investigators and guarantors

Contents

Contributors

Hermann Brenner
German Cancer Research Center
Division of Clinical Epidemiology
and Aging Research
Bergheimer Str. 20
69115 Heidelberg, Germany

Alarcos Cieza
ICF Research Branch of WHO CC
FIC (DIMDI), Institute for Health and
Rehabilitation Sciences (IHRS)
Ludwig-Maximilian University
Marchioninistr. 17
81377 Munich, Germany
Alarcos.Cieza@med.uni-muenchen.de

Linda Davies
Health Methodology Research Group
University of Manchester
Oxford Road
Manchester M13 9PL, UK
linda.davies@manchester.ac.uk

Paul Dieppe
Medical Research Council
Health Services Research Collaboration
Department of Social Medicine
University of Bristol
Canynge Hall, Whiteladies Road
Bristol BS8 2 PR, UK
P.Dieppe@bristol.ac.uk

Daniel Dornacher
Department of Orthopedics
Ulm University
Oberer Eselsberg 45
89081 Ulm, Germany
Daniel.dornacher@uni-ulm.de

Maxime Dougados
René Descartes University
Assistance Publique – Hôpitaux de Paris
Cochin Hospital
27 rue du Faubourg Saint Jacques
75014 Paris
France
m.doug@cch.ap-hop-paris.fr

Karsten Dreinhöfer
Department of Orthopedics
Ulm University
Oberer Eselsberg 45
89081 Ulm
Germany
karsten.dreinhoefer@uni-ulm.de

Markus Flören
Department of Orthopedics
Ulm University
Oberer Eselsberg 45
89081 Ulm
Germany
markus.floeren@uni-ulm.de

Klaus-Peter Günther
Department of Orthopedics
Universitätsklinikum Carl Gustav Carus
Fetscherstr. 74
01307 Dresden
Germany
Klaus-Peter.Guenther@
uniklinikum-dresden.de

Olof Johnell
Department of Orthopaedics
Faculty of Medicine
Malmö University Hospital
205 02 Malmö

Peter Jüni
Institute of Social and Preventive Medicine
Universität Bern
Finkenhubelweg 11
3012 Bern
Switzerland
juni@ispm.unibe.ch

Thomas Kohlmann
Institute for Community Medicine
Ernst Moritz Arndt Universität Greifswald
Walther-Rathenau-Str. 48
17487 Greifswald
Germany
thomas.kohlmann@uni-greifswald.de

Martin Krismer
Department of Orthopedics,
Medical University of Innsbruck
Anichstrasse 35
A-6020 Innsbruck
Austria
martin.krismer@uibk.ac.at

S. Lohmander
Department of Orthopedics
Lund University
Lund University Hospital
22185 Lund,
Sweden
stefan.lohmander@med.lu.se

Dagmar Lühmann
Institute for Social Medicine,
University of Lübeck
Beckergrube 43-47
23552 Lübeck
Germany
dagmar.luehmann@uk-sh.de

Henrike Merx
Landratsamt Rems-Murr-Kreis
Kreishaus Waiblingen, Germany
h.merx@arcor.de

Anna Nilsdotter
Department of Research and
Education
Halmstad Central Hospital
301 85 Halmstad,
Sweden
Anna.Nilsdotter@lthalland.se

Wolfhart Puhl
University of Ulm
Oberer Eselsberg
89081 Ulm
Germany
wolfhart.puhl@efort.org

Heiko Reichel
Department of Orthopedics
Ulm University
Oberer Eselsberg 45
89081 Ulm
Germany
heiko.reichel@uniklinik-ulm.de

Götz Röderer
Department of Trauma, Hand- and
Reconstructive Surgery
Ulm University
Oberer Eselsberg 45
89081 Ulm
Germany
goetz.roederer@uniklinik-ulm.de

Caroline Sanders
National Primary Care Research and
Development Centre
The University of Manchester
Williamson Building, Oxford Road
Manchester M13 9PL,
UK
caroline.sanders@manchester.ac.uk

Peter Schräder
Orthopädische Universitätsklinik
Mannheim
Theodor-Kutzer-Ufer 1-3
68167 Mannheim
Germany

Uwe Schütz
Department of Orthopedics
Department of Diagnostic and
Interventional Radiology
Ulm University
Oberer Eselsberg
89081 Ulm
Germany
uwe.schuetz@uniklinik-ulm.de

Gerold Stucki
Department of Physical Medicine and
Rehabilitation
University Hospital Munich
Marchioninistr.15
81377 Munich,
Germany
gerold.stucki@med.uni-muenchen.de

Til Stürmer
Harvard Medical School
Brigham and Women's Hospital Division
of Pharmacoepidemiology
and Pharmacoeconomics
1620 Tremont Street
Suite 3030, Boston
MA 02120,
USA
til.sturmer@post.harvard.edu

Wilfried von Eiff
Institut für Krankenhausmanagement
Westfälische Wilhelms-Universität
Münster
Centrum für Krankenhaus-Management
Röntgenstr. 9, 48149 Münster
Germany
ckm@wiwi.uni-muenster.de

Jack I. Williams
Institute for Clinical Evaluative Sciences
2075 Bayview Avenue
Toronto, ON
Canada M4N 3M5

Gilian Woolhead
Medical Research Council
Health Services Research Collaboration
Department of Social Medicine
University of Bristol
Canynge Hall
Whiteladies Road
Bristol BS8 2 PR
UK
gillian.woolhead@bristol.ac.uk

Dominik Ziegler
Department of Orthopedics
Ulm University
Oberer Eselsberg 45
89081 Ulm
Germany
dominik.ziegler@uni-ulm.de

Introduction: The Provision of Hip Joint Replacement

Karsten Dreinhöfer, Klaus-Peter Günther, Paul Dieppe, and Wolfhart Puhl

In their Preface to this book, the responsible investigators outlined why and how they set up the "Eurohip" project. Having secured the interest of a large group of orthopaedic surgeons and health services researchers from many parts of Europe, they needed to bring them together to discuss what key projects they should be undertake. We, the editors of this book, were charged with organising a meeting to help fulfil that aim.

The meeting was held in the Hotel Sonnenalp, Ofterschwang, Germany in June 2000. It was attended by colleagues from Canada and other countries with expert knowledge and experience in research on the provision of hip replacement, in addition to members of the Eurohip group. Several presentations were made, and the excellent discussions that followed helped facilitate the development of Eurohip's core projects.

Those attending thought that the meeting's proceedings were worthy of publication, so after the conclusion of the meeting we asked the presenters if they would prepare a manuscript for us. We were delighted when nearly all of them agreed. Furthermore, when we gave them the opportunity to update their work in the light of the delay between the time of the meeting and publication of this book, most of the contributors graciously agreed to do that. This book is the outcome of their labours, for which we are most grateful.

The individual chapters cover some of the main problems and unanswered questions about the provision of total hip joint replacement. The topics covered include the evidence for practice variations, aspects of the indications for total joint replacement, including patient perspectives, economic issues and outcome assessment.

Many of the authors have separately published the work reported here in scientific journals, but by bringing these contributions together in a single publication we hope that we have been able to provide interested readers with a clearer overview of the subject. Recent surveys of the literature suggest to us that the time delay has not affected the relevance of these chapters to current health care provision.

K. Dreinhöfer (✉)
Department of Orthopedics, Ulm University, Oberer Eselsberg 45, 89081 Ulm, Germany
e-mail: karsten.dreinhoefer@uni-ulm.de

K.E. Dreinhöfer et al. (eds.), *EUROHIP: Health Technology Assessment of Hip Arthroplasty in Europe*, DOI: 10.1007/978-3-540-74137-4_1, © 2009 EFORT

1

As we bring this book to publication we are in the middle of the WHO's "Bone and Joint Decade". The "Decade" is trying to increase awareness and understanding of bone and joint diseases. The Eurohip project is proud to be a part of that movement and we are delighted that the leaders of the "Decade" have agreed to the proceedings of our initial meeting being published as part of their work.

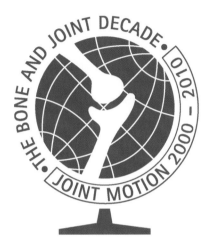

Part I

**Health Technology Assessment
of Hip Arthoplasty**

International Variations in Hip Replacement Rates*

2

H. Merx, P. Schräder, T. Stürmer, K. Dreinhöfer,
W. Puhl, K.-P. Günther, and H. Brenner

2.1
Introduction

Radiographically-defined osteoarthritis (OA) of the hip affects about 15% of individuals over 65 years old in countries with Caucasian populations [1–3]. Hip OA can lead to pain and impaired function, and is known to be an important cause of disability in later life. Total direct and indirect costs of musculoskeletal diseases, of which arthritis is an important subcategory, have risen in the last 15 years, accounting for up to 1–3.5% of the gross national product in countries like Australia, Canada, the United States or the United Kingdom [4–7].

A number of studies have shown that total hip replacement (THR) effectively relieves symptoms of advanced hip OA and restores the loss of function [8–11]. In addition, THR is cost effective compared to other treatment options [12, 13]. Despite its major role in treatment of OA, different indication criteria to THR seem to be applied. The aim of our study was to sample health utilisation data for THR in the countries of the developed world, especially OECD countries (Organisation for Economic Co-operation and Development) and to investigate whether missing consensus criteria result in different replacement rates.

*Originally publication: H. Merx, K.E. Dreinhöfer, P. Schräder, T. Stürmer, W. Puhl, K.-P. Günther, H. Brenner. International variation in hip replacement rates Annals of Rheumatic Diseases 2003; 63 (3): 222–226

H. Merx (✉)
Landratsamt Rems-Murr-Kreis, Kreishaus Waiblingen, Germany
h.merx@arcor.de

2

2.2
Methods

To obtain national THR rates we compiled data from the available literature, different data sources of national authorities and finally information from hip implant manufacturers. For information on further country-specific indicators, such as the population age structure or general health care costs, we also used the OECD Health Data File 1999.

2.2.1
Literature Review

MEDLINE searches were performed for the period 1990–2000. We used "total hip arthroplasty", "total hip replacement", "total hip implant", "THA" combined with "incidence", "population-based", "osteoarthritis" as search terms. Only articles in English, German or Dutch languages were considered. Further bibliographies and cross-referencing of identified papers were used for completion of the study.

The review includes only population-based studies with a specified data source of performed THR. In most cases, the data source was either a national register or the hospital records/operating theatre registers of an entire country, county or smaller area. Publications with district data were only included in the study in the absence of national data. Moreover, national or district THR rates were only considered if the reference population was the total population. If there were several publications pertaining to the same data source, e.g. a national register, only the most recent one was taken into consideration.

Whenever possible, the THR rates as provided in the publications were used. In some cases, only numbers of THR units were given in the publications. In these cases, the OECD-Health-Data File 1999 was the data source for the population to calculate THR rates. With few exceptions, only crude rather than age-specific or age-standardized THR rates are presented since only very few THR figures by age groups were recorded.

2.2.2
Information from National Authorities

In order to get information on national data of THR rates we performed a survey among national authorities. We asked, in a standardised questionnaire, for annual rates, or, alternatively, absolute numbers of primary THR and overall hip replacements (sum out of primary THR, partial hip replacement and hip revision procedures) for the years 1985, 1990, 1995 and the most recent year with available data. As OA is a major diagnosis for THR, we also asked for hospitalisation rates due to OA (ICD-9: 715). Additionally, we requested further information on the data source (i.e. the coding system, National Register, percentage of the

National Hospitals) and, if available, more detailed data such as age- or sex-specific hospitalisation rates.

This questionnaire was sent to national authorities of all OECD countries except Korea and Mexico, since no pertinent addresses could be identified in those countries. Additionally we got in touch with organisations in Singapore as a developed Asian country. Beside National Statistical Offices, National Health Ministries and other relevant national authorities were searched by Internet. We also contacted all organisations as indicated by those mentioned above; overall more than 90 institutions in 30 countries. Non-responders were sent a maximum of two reminders.

Official data on hospitalisation due to THR and/or OA rates were obtained from 23 countries. Data from two countries (Greece, Luxembourg) were not available in the requested form, while authorities from one country required a prohibitive charge. The contacted institutions of four countries (Belgium, Italy, Netherlands, Turkey) reported a lack of access to the requested data. Swiss data had to be excluded because they may not be representative for the country. Only 50% of the Swiss hospitals reported data to the authorities before 1996.

Crude hospitalisation rates were calculated by relating annual numbers of events with population figures of the OECD Health-Data-File 99 if necessary. The most recent year for which population figures were available in this data source was 1997, and the 1997 figures were also used to calculate approximate rates for more recent years (1998, 1999).

2.2.3
Information of Hip Implant Manufacturers

We asked seven leading manufacturers of hip implants for information of the hip joint replacement market in Europe, North America and in some Pacific countries. We received the requested data from four companies (Aesculap, Biomet, De Puy, Sulzer). Generally, these computations were based on several data sources such as information from industry participants, key academic conferences, national orthopaedic associations, statistical offices, market literature or market intelligence services The majority of data pertained to "hip implant units" without further specification on primary THR, partial hip replacement or revision procedures. Numbers of hip implants were again combined with population figures from the OECD Health-Data-File 1999 to estimate crude implantation rates.

Manufacturing companies' data of national hip implant rates were only included in this survey if they covered the period 1997–1999 and if at least data of two companies for one country were available.

National authorities in different countries and international orthopaedic companies do not always record the same data type. To demonstrate as much relevant information as possible, we present two end-point criteria, national THR rates and overall national hip implantation rates. The latter summarise THR, partial hip replacement and hip revision procedures.

2.3
Results

2.3.1
Country-Specific Primary THR Rates

2.3.1.1
Review of the Literature

Published crude annual primary THR rates for Caucasian people vary between 50/100,000 and 125/100,000 inhabitants (Table 2.1). For the period since 1990, the annual THR rates were reported to be between 100 and 125 in Norway [14], Iceland [15], Sweden [16] and the Netherlands [17], whereas for England [18], Australia [3] and the western part of Scotland [19], the corresponding rate varied between 65 and 90. For some countries, only earlier data were available. In the period 1988–1990, the crude annual THR rate in Denmark was 82/100,000 [20], in Finland 58/100,000 [21], in Canada 50/100,000 [22] and in Olmsted County (Minnesota, USA) 60/100,000 [23]. A study of ethnic groups within the cosmopolitan population of San Francisco (California, USA) showed large ethnic differences in the incidence of THR [24]. THR rates for whites were two to ten times higher than those of any other ethnic group (Black, Hispanics, Asians). For the residents of Maryland (USA), the annual THR rate was reported to be 59/100,000 in the years 1985–1987 with a black to white ratio of 0.73 [25].

As shown in Table 2.1, primary OA is the main indication for more than 65% of all primary THRs performed in the Scandinavian countries, Scotland and Australia. In different ethnic groups of San Francisco, the proportion of OA among indications of THR varies between ethnic groups. The highest proportion was found for white people (66%), followed by black people (55%), Hispanics (54%), and Asians (<29%). Among Japanese men and women living in Hawaii, only 30% and 36% of all THR were performed because of OA [26].

Below the age of 50 years, THR rates we re very low and quite similar for all ethnic groups of Hawaii (White, Japanese, Chinese, Hawaiians, Filipino) [26]. For those older than 50, the white population has markedly higher THR rates than the other ethnic groups (see Fig. 2.1). The age-specific THR rate of white persons increases steadily up to 75–79 years and declines thereafter (see Fig. 2.2). These observations from England and the United States are consistent with data in western/northern European countries and in Canada [15, 18, 23, 27].

2.3.1.2
National Health Authorities Data

According to information of the contacted national authorities, the crude national (primary) THR rate in 1998 varied between 8 and 135/100,000 inhabitants (Table 2.2). France and the Scandinavian countries reported a high rate of primary THR with about 90 procedures per 100,000 inhabitants. Markedly lower rates were registered in Ireland with 63 primary THR/100,000 inhabitants and in the United States with 53 primary THR/100,000

Table 2.1 Annual primary THR rates/100,000 inhabitants – literature data

	Period	Annual primary THR rate (per 100,000)	Done for OA (%)	Data source	Reference
Norway	1995–1998	110–120	68[a]	National register	Havelin [14]
Iceland	1992–1996	114*	68	Records of all orthopaedic clinics	Ingvarsson et al. [15]
England	1995–1996	78[b]	49[c]–84[d]	Hospital episode system (NHS hospitals)	Birrell et al. [18]
Australia	1997–1998	72	>90[e]	National registry	Williamson [3]
The Netherlands	1994	105		SIG Zorginformatie (total population)	Okhuijsen et al. [17]
Sweden	1991–1995	108–125	76[f]	National register	Herberts and Malchau [16]
Scotland (west of Scotland)	1/9/1991 - 28/2/1993	67[g] (urban) 86[g] (rural)	86 (urban) 89 (rural)	Hospital records of all 16 hospitals in the west of Scotland	Dunsmuir et al. [19]
Canada	1/4/1988 - 31/3/1990	50*,[h]		Canadian hospital morbidity file	Gentleman et al. [22]
USA (San Francisco)	1984–1988	White: 76*,[i] Black: 35*,[i] Hispanics: 13*,[i] Asians: <17*,[i]	White: 66 Black: 55 Hispanics: 54 Asians: <29	Hospital records of the 17 hospitals within or near San Francisco	Hoaglund et al. [24]

(continued)

Table 2.1 (continued)

	Period	Annual primary THR rate (per 100,000)	Done for OA (%)	Data source	Reference
USA Olmsted County (Minnesota)	1987–1990	60[j]	ca 75	Registry of the Mayo Clinic, data of the Rochester Epidemiology Project	Madhock et al. [23]
Denmark (South Jutland)	1988–1990	82	86 (1981–1990)	Hospital records of the two orthopaedic hospitals in South Jutland	Overgaard et al. [20]
Finland	1988	58	71[k]	National register	Paavolainen et al. [21]
USA (Maryland)	1985–1987	59*		Hospital discharges in Maryland	Gittelsohn et al. [25]

*Total hip replacement procedures

[a] Data source: Havelin et al. [29]

[b] Data source: Hospital Episode System [all patients admitted to hospitals of the National Health Service (NHS), including private patients treated in NHS Hospitals]

[c] Data for 1989 [18]

[d] 84% of all elective THRs done for OA in six districts of the Oxford region [30]

[e] Data from a Registry pilot study of 260 patients undergoing a primary THR or a primary total knee replacement

[f] Data source: Herberts and Malchau [31]

[g] Age- and sex-standardised rates to the Scottish population, primary elective THR

[h] CCP code 93.5

[i] Age-standardised rates to the 1986-specific racial population

[j] Age-and sex-standardised rates to the population structure of US whites in 1980

[k] Reference to all (hip, knee, other) arthroplastiesv

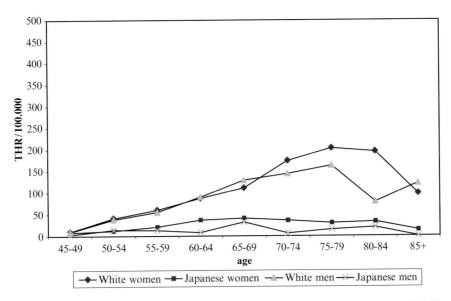

Fig. 2.1   Age- and sex-specific THR rates per 100,000 inhabitants – ethnic groups of Hawaii [26]

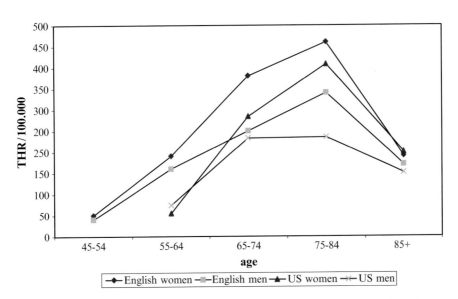

Fig. 2.2   Age- and sex-specific THR rates/100,000 inhabitants – England [28] and USA [32]

inhabitants. Only 8 THR/100,000 inhabitants were reported for Singapore. The reported THR rates from Hungary and Singapore do not permit a further differentiation between primary and revision arthroplasty procedures. Therefore, primary THR rates are likely to be slightly lower for these countries.

   In the last decade, differences in the development of the national annual THR rates are observable. Whereas in Norway and Sweden, countries with a high THR rate in 1990, the

Table 2.2 Annual primary THR rates/100,000 inhabitants – national health authorities data

	1985 or the next later year	1990 or the next later year	1995 or the next later year	1998	Procedure	Data source/sector
Australia		61		73	Primary THR	Public and most private hospitals
Denmark	70	74		90	Primary THR[a]	National register
England		55	68	71	Primary THR[b]	Public hospitals[c]
Finland	44	66	88	93	Primary THR[*]	National register
France				135	Primary THR[d]	Public and private hospitals
Hungary			51	70[+]	THR[e]	No information
Iceland	62	66	79	90[+]	Primary THR for OA	Records of all orthopaedic clinics
Ireland			72	63	Primary THR[f]	Public hospitals
Norway	95	114	117	121	Primary THR	National register
Scotland		47	74	81	Primary THR[b]	Public hospitals
Singapore			6	8	THR[*]	All hospitals
Sweden	106	102	108	118	Primary THR[g]	National register
United States			51	53[§]	Primary THR[f]	Non-federal hospitals
Wales			78	69	Primary THR[b]	Public hospitals

[*]We did not receive further information on the coding system

[+]1999

[§]1997

[a]The classification of surgical procedures has changed in 1988 and 1996

[b]OPCS4: W371, W381, W391

[c]All patients admitted to NHS hospitals, including private patients treated in NHS Hospitals

[d]W795, W436-W440, W451

[e]International Classification of Procedures, WHO, 1978, 58150–58153, 5815A,B,D-F

[f]ICD-9-CM: 81.51 (total hip replacement)

[g]ICD-9: 8410 + 8414, ICD-10; NFB2 + NFB3 + NFB4

annual primary THR rate increased only slightly between 1990 and 1998, the Scottish and Finnish rates which were low in 1990 increased by 70% and 40% during this period, respectively.

2.3.2
Country Specific Overall Hip Implantation Rates

2.3.2.1
National Health Authorities Data

For overall hip implantation, defined as THR, partial hip replacement and hip revision procedures combined, for 1998 the national authorities reported crude rates between 27 and 192 operations per 100,000 inhabitants (see Table 2.3). In accordance with the primary THR data, the French rate was the highest one with 192 hip implants/100,000 inhabitants, whereas in most other western and northern European countries 100–150 hip implant procedures/100,000 inhabitants were performed. Lower national hip replacement rates were reported from eastern European countries and from Portugal. With less than 30 hip implantations/100,000 persons, the inhabitants of Singapore and the Pacific people of New Zealand had the lowest hip implantation rates.

The large national differences in the relationship of total to partial hip replacement procedures are remarkable in this context. In Hungary, for example, this ratio is reported to be 10:1, in Australia nearly 3:1, in England 2:1, in the United States of America slightly over 1:1 and in Singapore 1:2.5 (data not shown).

As the Norwegian data do not include the hemiprostheses and the Polish and the Portuguese data do not include the hip revision procedures, the reported implant numbers of these countries are likely to underestimate the hip replacement procedures actually performed.

2.3.2.2
Information of Hip Implant Manufacturers

According to business data, Switzerland, France and Germany have worldwide the highest hip implantation rates (Table 2.4). Estimations of country-specific hip implantation rates vary between 100–160 procedures per 100,000 inhabitants for many northern and western European countries, while 60–100 hip procedures per 10^5 inhabitants were reported for southern European countries and for the United States, followed by Japan with 45–74 hip implants/100,000 inhabitants.

2.3.3
Country Specific OA Rates

The reported annual hospital discharge rates for OA varied between 200 and 320 discharges/100,000 inhabitants in 1995 or later for most of the western and northern European countries and for some eastern European countries like Hungary and the Czech Republic.

2

Table 2.3 Annual hip implantation rates/100,000 inhabitants – national health authorities data

	1985 or the next later year	1990 or the next later year	1995 or the next later year	1998	Procedure	Data source/sector
Australia				117	THR, partial hip replacements and revision procedures*	Public and most private hospitals
Denmark	72	121	125	146	[a]	National register
England		115	128	137	[b]	Public hospitals~
Finland		109	133	145	Hip replacements*	National register
France				192	[c]	Public and private hospitals
Hungary			57	78+	[d]	No information
Ireland			110	107	[e]	Public hospitals
New Zealand				80§,°	Hip replacements*	Public hospitals
Norway	110	131	140	145	Primary and revision THR[f]	National register
Poland	28	31	35		[g]	Central hospital register
Portugal			41	60+	Total and partial hip replacements[h]	Public hospitals
Singapore			23	27+	Hip implantations[j]	All hospitals
Sweden	129	127	136	151	[j]	National register
United States			99	102#	[e]	Non-federal hospitals
Wales			151	139	[b]	Public hospitals

* We did not receive further information on the coding system

~ All patients admitted to NHS hospitals, including private patients treated in NHS Hospitals

+ 1999, § 1997, # 1996

° Standardised discharge ratio (ratio of observed to expected discharge rates – age/gender standardised) of pacific people: 0.3

[a] 1998: NFB, NFC Nomesco classification of surgical procedures 1990/1995: 70030–39, 70230–39, 70130–39, 70330–39 1985: 8270, 8274

[b] OPCS4: W37-W39, W46-W48

[c] W435-W454, W795

[d] International Classification of Procedures, WHO, 1978: 58150–58159, 5815A–F, 58169

[e] ICD-9-CM: 81.51, 81.52, 81.53

[f] Hemiprostheses not recorded

[g] 5-820

[h] ICD-9-CM: 81.51, 81.52

[i] Total and partial hip replacement, for hip revision procedures no detailed information available

[j] ICD-9: 8410, 8413–15, 8419, NFB0–4, NFB9, NFC

Table 2.4 Information of hip implant manufacturers

	Hip implants/100,000 inhabitants[a]
Austria	164–172
Belgium	158–160
France	162–201
Germany	145–183
Italy	66–90
Japan	45–74
Netherlands	115–119
Norway	145–146
Spain	62–102
Sweden	113–145
Switzerland	200–206
UK	101–132
United States	75–109

[a]Range of estimates from four companies

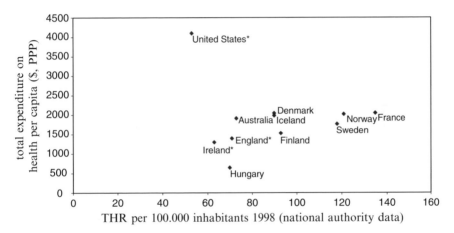

Fig. 2.3 THR/100,000 inhabitants and total expenditure on health/capita in OECD countries

Higher rates were reported for Austria and Finland with more than 400 discharges/100,000 inhabitants, and lower rates (100–150 discharges/100,000 inhabitants) for the United States, New Zealand and Poland. Fewer than 100 discharges due to OA/100,000 inhabitants were registered in Portugal, Spain, Japan and Singapore in 1995.

2.3.4
Country-Specific General Health Care Costs

In 1997, total expenditure on health per capita (purchasing power parity) varied between $400 and $4,000 (all amounts in US dollars) (Fig. 2.3). By far the highest expenditures on health were reported for the United States with $4,095 per capita, followed by Switzerland

($2,611) and Germany ($2,364). Most Scandinavian countries and some western European countries like France, The Netherlands and Belgium spent between $1,750 and $2,050, while New Zealand, the United Kingdom and most southern European countries spent between $1,000 and $1,500. Less than $1,000 were spent in 1997 in eastern European OECD countries.

2.4
Discussion

THR is a common orthopaedic procedure in the elderly. However, detailed epidemiologic data on frequency of hip replacement is rare. We therefore collected all available country-specific hip replacement data for the OECD countries using different data sources.

Rates of THR varied considerably between the contacted OECD countries with a predominantly Caucasian population. The crude national annual THR rates as reported by National Authorities varied between 50 and 140 procedures/100,000 inhabitants. These data are consistent with publications based on hospital records or on administrative data sources [3, 14–20, 23]. As most data come from Scandinavian or English-speaking countries, the variation of crude THR rates may even be greater between all of the OECD countries. The reported low hip implantation rates for Poland and Portugal, the very low Spanish and Portuguese hospital discharge rates with the diagnosis of OA and the low business data for hip implantation procedures in Italy and Spain may be indications for relative low THR rates in some eastern and southern European countries. High computations of several companies for the hip implant market in Switzerland and Germany in combination with the high total expenditure on health per capita in these countries may indicate high primary THR rates.

Caucasian men and women have substantially higher THR rates than all other ethnic groups. The low THR rates of Asian people living in San Francisco and Hawaii [24, 26] are consistent with the reported low national THR rates of Singapore residents and the low hip implantation rate of the Pacific people of New Zealand, indicating different prevalence rates for OA in different ethnic groups. However, other factors such as differential access to health care by ethnicity may also play a role.

Although we attempted to acquire comparable data for each country, this was not always possible, because of different types of documentation systems in national authorities, orthopaedic societies and implant manufacturers. Other sources of restrictions and uncertainties were different national coding systems, the scarcity of information about procedures performed in the private health care sector, uncertainty regarding data quality in terms of completeness, comparability over time, etc. So even when comparing one single procedure, for example primary THR, the compilation of comparative data within different countries is difficult.

Most national primary THR rates are based on different coding systems. The three-digit ICD-9-CM-code, which is used for example in the United States and in Ireland, allows differentiation of THR, partial hip replacement and hip revision. The specification of the French coding system, which is derived from the American DRG, or of the OPCS4 code used in England, Scotland and Wales, is more detailed. In consequence, reported THR rates of some countries include, for example, terms such as unspecified hip procedures while others do not. Furthermore, no detailed information on hip revisions is available for Singapore and Hungary, so that the reported THR data of these countries probably include the revision procedures.

Additionally, the variety of information about procedures performed in the private health care sector also influences national THR rates. Singapore with a central claims processing system, the Scandinavian countries with National Hip Arthroplasty Registries and France with the recently installed Medical Information System include public as well as private hospitals in their statistics. However, for many other countries, the completeness of the data has to be questioned. In England, the Hospital Episode Statistics, which is the data source of the reported THR rates, covers all patients treated in hospitals of the National Health Service (NHS) and includes private insurance payment. However, additionally to the reported 32,800 primary THR performed in NHS Hospitals, about 11,000 THR procedures are carried out in the private sector [28]. Similarly, the reported hip implantation data of Portugal and New Zealand refer only to the National Service Hospitals without further information on the THR procedures performed in private institutions. Consequently, the true incidence of THR or of hip implantations is underestimated in these countries.

As the age-specific THR incidence steadily increases in Caucasian people with age from 50 up to 75–79 years and declines thereafter, age-standardised incidence rates are needed for a direct comparison between populations in order to eliminate differences in country-specific age structures. OECD-countries with a relative young population – defined as less than 12% of the total population being older than 65 years in 1997 – are Iceland, Ireland, Poland, New Zealand and Australia. OECD countries with a relative "old" population – defined as more than 15% of the total population being older than 65 years – are, for example, Sweden, the United Kingdom, France, and Norway. Ingvarsson et al. [15] demonstrated the implications of different population age structures by comparing Swedish and Icelandic THR rates. On the basis of crude incidence rates, there seemed to be no difference between both countries, but after age standardisation THR incidence was at least 50% higher in Iceland than in Sweden. In the present paper, we were unfortunately unable to perform an age-standardisation because the few age-specific THR data obtainable were based on different age-strata. Comparisons between countries with different age structures should therefore be interpreted with caution.

Besides limitations regarding the completeness and the comparability of the data, differences in the economic structure may also influence national THR rates. In 1997, great differences in total expenditure on health per capita ($ purchasing power parity) were reported in OECD countries. Countries with high expenditure on health often tended to have higher THR rates than countries with low expenditure. But whereas low expenditure on health indeed seems to be an important cause for low national THR rates, high expenditure on health does not always correlate with high THR rates as the French, Norwegian and Danish data demonstrate. Having comparable high expenditure on health per capita and a similar population age structure, great national differences in THR procedures per 100,000 inhabitants were observed in these countries. Comparatively few THR procedures were also performed in the United States and in Canada, two of the five countries with the

2

highest expenditure on health, even with regard to the relative young population age structure.

Despite these limitations, our results indicate major variation in hip replacement rates between developed countries which is unlikely to be explained by different economic structures, by differences in OA rates or age structure of the populations studied alone, and which underline the need of commonly agreed indication criteria.

Acknowledgement Dr. H. Merx was supported by the Bertelsmann Foundation within the project "Degenerative Joint Disease".

References

1. Sun Y, Stürmer T, Günther K, Brenner H. Inzidenz und Prävalenz der Cox- und Gonarthrose in der Allgemeinbevölkerung. Z Orthop 1997;135:184–192.
2. Ingvarsson T, Hägglund G, Lohmander LS. Prevalence of hip osteoarthritis in Iceland. Ann Rheum Dis 1999;58:201–201.
3. Williamson OW. Measuring the success of joint replacement surgery. Med J Aust 1999;171:229–230.
4. Badley EM. The economic burden of musculoskeletal disorders in Canada is similar to that for cancer, and may be higher. J Rheumatol 1995;22:204–206.
5. Coyte PC, Asche CV, Croxford R, Chan B. The economic cost of musculoskeletal disorders in Canada. Arthritis Care Res 1998;11:315–325.
6. March LM, Bachmeier CJM. Economics of osteoarthritis: a global perspective. Baillieres Clin Rheumatol 1997;11:817–834.
7. Yelin E, Callahan LF. The economic cost and social and psychological impact of musculoskeletal conditions. National Arthritis Data Work Groups. Arthritis Rheum 1995;38:1351–1362.
8. Bachmeier CJ, March LM, Cross MJ, Lapsley HM, Tribe KL, Courtenay BG, et al. A comparison of outcomes in osteoarthritis patients undergoing total hip and knee replacement surgery. Osteoarthritis Cartilage 2001;9:137–146.
9. Jones CA, Voaklander DC, Johnston DW, Suarez-Almazor ME. Health related quality of life outcomes after total hip and knee arthroplasties in a community based population. J Rheumatol 2000;27:1745–1752.
10. Tate D, Sculco TP. Advances in total hip arthroplasty. Am J Orthop 1998;27:274–282.
11. Towheed TE, Hochberg MC. Health-related quality of life after total hip replacement. Semin Arthritis Rheum 1996;26:483–491.
12. Hirsch HS. Total joint replacement: a cost-effective procedure for the 1990s. Med Health R I 1998;81:162–164.
13. Chang RW, Pellisier JM, Hazen GB. A cost-effectiveness analysis of total hip arthroplasty for osteoarthritis of the hip. JAMA 1996;275:858–865.
14. Havelin LI. The Norwegian joint registry. Bull Hosp Jt Dis 1999;58:139–147.
15. Ingvarsson T, Hägglund G, Jonsson H, Lohmander LS. Incidence of total hip replacement for primary osteoarthrosis in Iceland 1982–1996. Acta Orthop Scand 1999;70:229–233.
16. Herberts P, Malchau H. How outcome studies have changed total hip arthroplasty practices in Sweden. Clin Orthop 1997;344:44–60.
17. Okhuijsen SY, Dhert WJA, Faro LMC, Schrijvers AJP, Verbout AJ. De totaleheupprothese in Nederland. Ned Tidschr Geneeskd 1998;142:1434–1438.
18. Birrell F, Johnell O, Silman A. Projectiong the need for hip replacement over the next three decades: influence of changing demography and threshold for surgery. Ann Rheum Dis 1999;58:569–572.

19. Dunsmuir RA, Allan DB, Davidson LAG. Increased incidence of primary total hip replace-ment in rural communities. BMJ 1996;313:1370.
20. Overgaard S, Knudsen HM, Hansen LN, Mossing N. Hip arthroplasty in Jutland, Denmark – Age and sex-specific incidences of primary operations. Acta Orthop Scand 1992;63:536–538.
21. Paavolainen P, Hämäläinen M, Mustonen H, Slätis P. Registration of arthroplasties in Finland. Acta Orthop Scand 1991;62:27–30.
22. Gentleman JF, Vayda E, Parsons GF, Walsh MN. Surgical rates in subprovincial areas across Canada: ranking of 39 procedures in order of variation. Can J Surg 1996;39:361–367.
23. Madhock R, Lewallen DG, Wallrichs SL, Ilstrup DM, Kurland RL, Melton LJ. Trends in the utilization of primary total hip arthroplasty, 1969 through 1990: a population-based study in Olmsted County, Minnesota. Mayo Clin Proc 1993;68:11–18.
24. Hoaglund FT, Oishi CS, Gialamas GG. Extreme variations in racial rates of total hip arthro-plasty for primary coxarthrosis: a population-based study in San Francisco. Ann Rheum Dis 1995;54:107–110.
25. Gittelsohn AM, Halpern J, Sanchez RL. Income, race, and surgery in Maryland. Am J Public Health 1991;81:1435–1441.
26. Oishi CS, Hoaglund FT, Gordon L, Ross PD. Total hip replacement rates are higher among Caucasians than Asians in Hawaii. Clin Orthop 1998;353:166–174.
27. Naylor CD, De Boer DP. Variations in selected surgical procedures and medical diagnosis by year and region. In: Goel V, Williams JI, Anderson GM, Blackstien-Hirsch P, Fooks C, Naylor CD (eds). Patterns of health care in Ontario. The ICES Practice Atlas, 2nd Edition. Ottawa: Canadian Medical Association, 1996:54–63.
28. Sheldon T, Eastwood A, Sowden A, Sharp. Total hip replacement. Effective Health Care 1996;2:1–12.
29. Havelin LI, Espehaug B, Vollset SE, Engesæter LB, Langeland N. The Norwegian arthro-plasty register. Acta Orthop Scand 1993;64:245–251.
30. Seagroatt V, Tan HS, Goldacre M, Bulstrode C, Nugent I, Gill L. Elective total hip replace-ment: incidence, emergency readmission rate, and postoperative mortality. BMJ 1991;303:1431–1435.
31. Herberts P, Malchau H. Long-term registration has improved the quality of hip replacement. Acta Orthop Scand 2000;71:111–121.
32. Praemer A, Furner S, Rice DP. Musculoskeletal conditions in the United States. American Academy of Orthopaedic Surgeons, 1999.

Health Technology Assessment of Hip Replacement

3

D. Lühmann

3.1
Background and Objectives

Osteoarthritis of the hip joint is a very common disorder among the elderly. In Germany, about 5% of the population above 60 years are suffering from symptomatic osteoarthritis of the hip. Typically, the disease is progressing slowly for years or even decades leading to a final state with severe pain and functional impairment of the affected joint. Consequently, the patients' quality of life is markedly diminished. During the 1960s, the development of prosthetic joint replacement led to a pivotal improvement of prognosis for these patients. Currently there are about 100,000 total hip replacements (THRs) performed per year in Germany in patients with osteoarthritis of the hip. Although the procedure yields satisfactory long-term results in 80–90% of cases, there is still a considerable amount of variability. Results may be influenced by patient characteristics (e.g. age, co-morbidity or compliance) by characteristics of the prosthetic device (e.g. material, method of fixation) or by details of the procedure itself (e.g. antimicrobial prophylactics, duration of the procedure, postoperative rehabilitation measures). For example: with respect to different types of prostheses 5-year failure rates between 0% and 20% are reported [1].

There were three main objectives for the following technology assessment:

1. To identify process and patient-related factors that determine outcomes after THR in patients with osteoarthritis either in a positive or negative direction. As far as process-related factors are concerned we were mainly interested in prosthesis type and fixation technique. Patient-related factors of interest were above all: age, weight and co-morbidities. As surrogate for successful surgery, we were interested in survival time of the prosthesis in situ and patient-related outcomes like pain, ability to walk, ability to perform activities of daily living and quality of life.

D. Lühmann (✉)
Institut für Sozialmedizin, Beckergrube 43-47, 23552, Lübeck, Germany

K.E. Dreinhöfer et al. (eds.), *EUROHIP: Health Technology Assessment of Hip Arthroplasty in Europe*, DOI: 10.1007/978-3-540-74137-4_3, © 2009 EFORT

2. The second objective was to describe current practice of THR surgery for osteoarthritis in Germany in terms of: indication and patient characteristics, prosthesis types and details of surgical procedure, as well as measures of peri- and postoperative care. As conclusions, we aimed to identify the potential for optimisation of current practice in order to improve outcomes.

3.2
Methods

Our technology assessment is based on data from a systematic analysis of the scientific literature. Taking into account the wealth of studies published on the subject, the search primarily focussed on: existing, recent Health Technology Assessment (HTA) Reports, systematic reviews and publications of arthroplasty registries. Recently published primary research was taken into consideration if, due to publication date or to the uniqueness of the topic (robotics), it was not included in the overviews. Publications were selected using predefined inclusion and exclusion criteria resulting from the objective formulated above:

- From the title or abstract of the review, HTA-report or guideline, it had to be obvious that the publication dealt with aspects addressed in our main objectives.
- The publication itself had to contain a systematic review of the literature.
- The language of the publication had to be English, German or Dutch or it had to include an abstract in English.

In order to be included, primary research publications had to fulfil the following criteria:

- At least 70% of the patient population with osteoarthritis
- Intervention: primary THR with specification of the prosthesis model
- Outcomes: clinical judgement of success (score or overall assessment, thigh pain), revision rates or need for revision (in addition: radiological signs of loosening)
- For controlled studies: at least 50 hips in each arm of the study, follow-up at least 5 years. For case series: at least 100 participants, follow-up at least 10 years

For assessment of methodological quality, we used checklists developed by the German Working Group Technology Assessment in Health Care in accordance with internationally accepted methodology (e.g. Cochrane Handbook). The instrument for assessment of HTA reports contains a section urging discussion of transferability of results to the German Health Care System. Finally, we performed a qualitative synthesis of the information.

To describe current practice of THR in Germany, we used two main sources of information. First, we obtained publications describing current practice of THR from the German scientific literature, accessed through electronic database searching as well as hand searching the relevant journals and websites. The second source of information was professional societies and renowned centres of excellence for osteoarthritis and orthopaedic surgery. These items of information were also compiled qualitatively.

3.3
Results

3.3.1
Review of the Literature

Five HTA reports [2–6], two reports from national implant registries [7, 8] and four systematic reviews [9–12] fulfilled the inclusion criteria. All overviews concluded that at the moment it is impossible to produce a conclusive summary of the literature that could serve as an evidence base to optimise THR. The main problems are the poor methodological quality of primary research, the multidimensionality of outcomes and the heterogeneity of instruments to measure them, the vast number of different prosthesis models available and finally the heterogeneous patient characteristics. The main body of research examines the influence of prosthesis model and fixation technique on revision rates (as a surrogate measure for failure). The best long-term (>20 years) survival rates are reported for older cemented prosthesis models (especially the model "Charnley"). Major improvements in survival rates were probably achieved by modification of cementing techniques. Up to now, revision rates of the Charnley are considered the "golden standard" which results of newly developed models should be measured against [e.g. 13]. Among the non-cemented prostheses, a few models yield comparably good results – but so far only for short and medium follow-up periods. Against this background, some authors [e.g. 3] suggest limiting the availability of prosthesis models in clinical practice and requiring proof of comparable effectiveness before marketing new models. Others [e.g. 2, 4, 5] recommend a close monitoring of results in THR surgery.

Concerning the influence of process-related details on postoperative results, the literature is not conclusive. The HTA-reports give no recommendations concerning these influences. In countries that run implant registries (Sweden, Norway and Finland), feedback of results to the operating centres seems to improve process quality (cementing technique, antibiotic prophylactics). The systematic reviews do not yield results that are readily transferable into clinical practice. A comparative review on antimicrobial prophylactics states that the efficacy of the new generation cephalosporins is not superior to that of the older generation [12]. Furthermore, there is no additional effect if therapy is extended beyond 24 h postoperatively. Another meta-analysis looking at the influence of prophylactic measure to prevent thromboembolism does not take all clinically relevant outcomes into account so the results are of little use to clinical practice [10]. Influences of patient characteristics (e.g. age, sex, co-morbidities, preoperative health status) are analysed in just a very limited number of studies. Interpretation of their results is complicated by interaction between different characteristics. At the moment it is not possible to draw firm conclusions on how to refine indications for hip replacement surgery with respect to different patient characteristics [11].

3

According to the authors of the HTA reports and systematic reviews, research needs to comprise above all:

- The development and implementation of a validated multidimensional set of instruments to assess outcomes of THR
- The comprehensive and country-specific documentation of clinical practice in THR
- Improvement of the methodological standard of evaluation studies

The literature search additionally retrieved 14 primary studies that fulfilled the inclusion criteria. They are not displayed in this context because their results just underlined the conclusions of the HTA reports presented above.

3.3.2
Current Practice of THR in Germany

Due to the lack of a standardised documentation system it is not possible to describe "state of the art of elective THR" in Germany. Specification of prosthesis models and implantation techniques used as well as peri- and postoperative supportive measures can only be described by exemplifying information from selected centres of excellence. Results from a few attempts of documentation (voluntary implant registries, surveys) are impaired by extremely low response rates [13–16]. But still, this very limited amount of information raises the suspicion that, in Germany, clinical practice THR is characterised by a large amount of heterogeneity and a tendency towards the implementation of innovative procedures. A survey performed as early as 1993 found 92 different prosthesis stems and 67 different cups (with different combinations of the two) resulting in hundreds of variants of implants being used in everyday clinical practice. Taking into account the literature available at the time, it was pointed out that prosthesis models with favourable long-term results were hardly in use in Germany.

The tendency towards innovation is furthermore demonstrated by the ongoing implementation of robot-assisted surgery into routine clinical practice in Germany – against a background of very limited evidence for efficacy and safety of the procedure (four studies [17–20] with a maximum of follow-up of 4 years). At the moment, it is not clear whether the patients will, compared to the results of conventional implantation techniques, experience net benefit or harm.

3.4
Conclusions

Outcomes of THR are influenced by a number of interacting factors. A systematic review of the scientific literature was not able to identify one or more factors that could be modified in order to improve outcomes of THR in general or in specific groups of patients.

Current practice of THR in Germany may only be described by exemplifying data from a few centres of excellence – it is probably characterised by a great amount of variability.

There is no comprehensive documentation system. The sparse information available suggests a tendency towards the implementation of new technologies into clinical practice without a base of sound scientific data on their efficacy.

In order to assure an adequate and high quality supply of THR surgery for patients with osteoarthritis, we suggest two prerequisites should be fulfilled:

1. Any strategy for improvement should be based on an exact documentation of current practice and its results. Ideally, not only structural and process-related information should be recorded but also a multidimensional description of the patients and their condition leading to surgery as well as its outcomes. The recommendation of the HTA reports cited above to implement comprehensive implant registries or a monitoring unit is supported.
2. Especially, data from the Scandinavian implant registries were able to show that influences of prosthesis model and implantation technique on long-term outcomes may sometimes become obvious only several years after surgery. Against this background, the continuous introduction of new prosthesis models into clinical practice leads to unforeseeable consequences for patients and operating surgeons. Therefore, it is suggested that,for new prosthesis models being marketed, there is a requirement for the submission of clinically relevant evidence of their equivalent or superior performance compared to standard models. If this type of evidence is not available, use of the device should be limited to the context of controlled trials. In the context of the German Health Care system, there are several pathways to put these recommendations into practice. First, the implementation of evidence-based guidelines may support transfer of scientific information into practice and at the same time point out the lack of evaluative research. Second, the regulative body for hospital care (Gemeinsamer Bundesausschuss) is, upon request, asked to judge against the background of scientific information whether a medical technology is needed to achieve sufficient, effective and efficient treatment of patients (covered by mandatory health insurance).

More systematic literature reviews are needed to further characterise the influence of perioperative measures, rehabilitation and patient-dependent characteristics, especially co-morbidity.

For the development of a standardised set of instruments for the documentation of THR results, an international effort seems necessary.

References

1. Lühmann D, Hauschild B, Raspe H: Hüftgelenkendoprothetik bei Osteoarthrose – Eine Verfahrensbewertung - Health Technology Assessment: Schriftenreihe des Deutschen Instituts für Medizinische Dokumentation und Information im Auftrage des Bundesministeriums für Gesundheit. Band 18. Nomos Verlagsgesellschaft Baden-Baden, 2000
2. Cowley DE: Prostheses for total hip replacement. Australian Institute for Health and Welfare, Health Care Technology Series, Number 12, February 1994
3. Sheldon T et al.: Total hip replacement. Nuffield Institute for Health, University of Leeds, NHS Center for Reviews and Dissemination: Effective Health Care 2(7); 1996

3

4. Faulkner A, Kennedy LG, Baxter K, Donovan J, Wilkinson M, Bevan G: Effectiveness of hip prostheses in primary total hip replacement: a critical review of evidence and an economic model. Health Technology Assessment 2(6); 1998
5. Fitzpatrick R, Shortall E, Sculpher M, Murray D, Morris R, Lodge M, Dawson J, Carr A, Britton A, Briggs A: Primary total hip replacement surgery: a systematic review of outcomes and modelling of cost-effectiveness associated with different prostheses. Health Technology Assessment 2(20); 1998
6. Pons JMV, Valls JM, Granados A: Effectiveness and efficiency in hip prosthesis surgery: elements for improvement. CAHTA, Barcelona, BR99006, 1999
7. Malchau H, Herberts P: Prognosis of total hip replacement. Revision and re-revision rate in THR: a revision-risk study of 148,359 primary operations. Scientific Exhibition presented at the 65th Annual Meeting of the American Academy of Orthopaedic Surgeons, March 19–23, 1998, New Orleans, USA
8. Espehaug B: Quality of total hip replacements in Norway 1987–1996. The Norwegian Arthroplasty Register. Bergen, Norway 1998
9. Towheed TE, Hochberg MC: Health-related quality of life after total hip replacement. Seminars in Arthritis and Rheumatism 26(1):483–491; August, 1996
10. Murray DW, Britton AR, Bulstrode CJK: Thromboprophylaxis and death after total hip replacement. From the Nuffield Orthopaedic Centre, Oxford, England; The Journal of Bone and Joint Surgery 78-B(6); November 1996
11. Young NL, Cheah D, Waddell JP, Wright JG: Patient characteristics that effect the outcome of total hip arthroplasty: a review. Canadian Journal of Surgery 41(3); June 1998
12. Glenny AM, Song F: Antimicrobial prophylaxis in total hip replacement: a systematic review. Health Technology Assessment 3(21); 1999
13. Gierse H, Maaz B, Wessolowski T: Hüft - Endoprothetik. Eine Standortbestimmung. Deutsches Ärzteblatt 89(42); 1992
14. Lang I, Buchhorn G, Willert HG: Hüftendoprothesensysteme in der Bundesrepublik Deutschland. Versuch einer Bestandsaufnahme. Orthopädie Mitteilungen 3:257–266; 1993
15. Kleimann H, Markefka B: Zusammenfassung der Potentialermittlung für Hüft- und Kniegelenkoperationen in Allgemeinkrankenhäusern der Bundesrepublik Deutschland. Orthopädie, Informationen BVO, Mitteilungen DGOT 5:445–448; 1996
16. Effenberger H, Mechtler R, Jerosch J, Munzinger U, Winter T: Qualitätssicherung in der Endoprothetik. Z Orthopädie 136:97–109; 1998
17. Bach CM, Winter P, Nogler M, Gobel G, Wimmer C, Ogon M: No functional impairment after Robodoc total hip arthroplasty: gait analysis in 25 patients. Acta Orthop Scand 73(4): 386–391; 2002
18. Okoniewski M, Birke A, Schietsch U, Thoma M, Hein W Z: Early results of a prospective study in patients with computer-assisted femur shaft preparation in total hip endoprosthesis implantation (Robodoc system) - indications, outcome, complications. Z Orthop Ihre Grenzgeb 138(6):510–514; 2000
19. Bargar WL, Bauer A, Borner M: Primary and revision total hip replacement using the Robodoc system. Clin Orthop 354:82–91; 1998
20. Borner M, Bauer A, Lahmer A: Computer-assisted robotics in hip endoprosthesis implantation. Unfallchirurg 100(8):640–645; 1997

The Economic Perspective on Joint Replacement and Equity

4

L. Davies

4.1
Introduction

Osteoarthritis is a major cause of hip or knee pain. The main treatment available is joint replacement, an effective and widely used but expensive intervention for which there are no evidence-based criteria for the indications or timing of these procedures [1]. Some smaller studies suggest no significant differences in outcome between age groups, obese and non-obese people, pre-operative functional status or underlying disease [2, 3]. In contrast, larger observational, registry databases and economic evaluations indicate that these factors plus level of social support and education are significant predictors of outcomes and of cost [4, 5]. Economic evaluation can provide a useful framework to analyse and interpret data to inform decisions about whether joint replacement should be available and who should be treated. The methods of economic evaluation are described in detail elsewhere [6]. This paper outlines some of the key issues that should be addressed by an economic evaluation.

4.2
How Does Economic Evaluation Define Whether Joint Replacement Is Worthwhile?

In general terms, a health care intervention is worthwhile if the value of the outcome, in terms of gains in health and social well-being, is greater than the value of the resources and services used to produce or provide that intervention. More specifically, if the decision has been made that treatment should be provided for a health condition, such as hip or knee pain, the question an economist asks is: What is the most efficient method of producing a gain in health and social well being for this condition? In this context, efficiency is defined as maximising the gain in health and social well-being associated with an intervention, such as a hip replacement, for a given budget.

L. Davies (✉)
Health Methodology Research Group, University of Manchester,
Oxford Road, Manchester, M13 9PL, UK
e-mail: linda.davies@manchester.ac.uk

K.E. Dreinhöfer et al. (eds.), *EUROHIP: Health Technology Assessment*
of Hip Arthroplasty in Europe, DOI: 10.1007/978-3-540-74137-4_4, © 2009 EFORT

4.3
What Should Joint Replacement Be Compared to?

Any economic evaluation to inform questions of technical efficiency requires that the intervention of interest, in this case joint replacement, is compared to an alternative. This is so that the additional or incremental costs and benefits of the joint replacement compared to the next best alternative can be assessed. The alternatives for comparison may include no joint replacement and usual care for the management of pain, reduced mobility, etc. An alternative may include more active intervention with physical therapy, manipulation or psychological therapy to manage or improve mobility and reduce the impact of pain, anxiety or distress.

4.4
Framework of Analysis

The main frameworks of analysis for economic evaluation are cost-effectiveness analysis, cost–utility analysis and cost–benefit analysis. All these frameworks require that there is a comparison of costs and outcomes between two or more interventions. The key difference is in the method of measuring and valuing outcomes. Cost-effectiveness analysis measures health gain using clinical outcome measures, such as life years gained or improvements in pain or in mobility. However, cost-effectiveness analyses do not combine different measures that are potentially important to patients and health care decision makers. For example, in the decision to provide a hip or knee replacement, surgeons and patients will need to trade the potential benefits of surgery against the risks of serious adverse events, such as surgical mortality, deep wound infection or failure of the prosthesis and the costs of the procedure. These aspects also need to be compared to the benefits, risks and costs of no surgery, or alternative interventions. The trade-offs of benefits and risks will be implicit if cost-effectiveness analysis is used to provide information about the relative value of joint replacement compared to available alternative interventions.

In contrast, cost–utility and cost–benefit analyses combine preferences for the matrix of benefits and risks that affect and health and social well-being into a single measure. Preferences for length of life and consequences, such as pain, reduced mobility, or infection that affect quality of life are combined by explicit trade-offs between each of these attributes. This allows the derivation of value weights that can be used to produce a summary measure of outcome. For example, consider (a) a year spent in full health with no problems. Compare this year of life to (b) a year spent with moderate pain or discomfort, no problems with walking about, self-care or usual activities and not feeling anxious or depressed, and to (c) a year of life spent in extreme pain or discomfort, with some problems in walking about, some problems with self-care and performing usual activities, and not being anxious or depressed. A typical ranking of these three health states would be state (a) full health as most preferred state, (b) as the next preferred option and state (c) as least preferred.

Now consider three additional health states: (d) a year of life spent with moderate pain or discomfort, some problems with walking about, self-care and usual activities and feeling extremely anxious or depressed whilst waiting for a hip or knee replacement; (e) a year

of life spent in extreme pain or discomfort, with some problems in walking about, no problems with self-care and performing usual activities and feeling moderately anxious or
depressed whilst waiting for a hip or knee replacement; and (f) immediate death due to
peri-operative complications during hip or knee surgery. The ranking of health states (a)–(f)
is not clear cut. For some people, full health (a) will be the most preferred and death (f) the
least preferred. For others, health states which include extreme pain or discomfort or
extreme anxiety or depression may be worse than death. The ranking and valuation of
health states that may occur also needs to consider the probability that they will or will not
occur. Consider an intervention where the probability of death (f) was 2% and the probability of full health was 98%. Compare this to an intervention where the probability of
death was 0% and the probability of health state (a) was 100%. Which would you prefer?
Cost–utility analysis and cost–benefit analysis seek to evaluate the trade-offs between
complex sets of benefits and risks by addressing the following questions. First, on average,
what is the order of preferences for health states (a)–(f) and second, by how much is one
health state preferred to another?

Cost–utility analysis uses a non-monetary measure of value, known as utility, to address
these questions. The utility weights are multiplied by length of life to produce a measure of
quality-adjusted life-years (QALYs). Cost–benefit analysis seeks to provide a monetary measure of the relative value of the different benefits and costs. The methods used to derive these
utility weights and the relative merits of the methods are described in detail elsewhere [6].

4.5
Whose Costs, Outcomes and Values Are Important in Choosing Joint Replacement?

From the economic perspective, an evaluation of the efficiency of an intervention should
include the costs of all resources used to provide care and all the outputs or consequences
of the intervention. This is termed the societal perspective and encompasses more limited
viewpoints, such as that of the hospital or secondary care sector responsible for providing
the joint replacement services, or the third party insurance system (public or private)
responsible for payment for the services used. Resources or services from a variety of sectors will be used as inputs to provide care and support prior to, during and after treatment.
Care after the intervention will include longer term follow-up and management and treatment for any adverse consequences as a result of the intervention.

In the case of hip or knee pain and joint replacement, these will include: first, primary
care services, such as GP visits for referral to secondary care or pain management; second,
community or social care to provide support, equipment and aids for reduced mobility or
problems in self-care and usual activities prior to joint replacement and rehabilitation
following the joint replacement; third, hospital inpatient and outpatient services to assess
the need for surgery and the patients suitability in terms of the risks and potential benefit
of a joint replacement, inpatient care for the joint replacement and post-surgical care, treatment
of adverse consequences of surgery, longer term follow-up and medication; and fourth, the
costs to the patient and family or friends in terms of time spent in care related activities and
additional expenditure. This may include time spent by the patient and carers to participate
in exercise programmes to regain mobility or lose weight before or after the operation and

4

time spent attending hospital services or other rehabilitation programmes. Both the patients and carers may incur additional expenditure, for travel costs, aids and adaptations to the home, social support or residential care and medication.

As noted above, the outputs will include benefits in terms of improved health and social well-being and also the impact of reduction health and social well-being associated with any adverse consequences of care. As with the inputs to care, the outputs to a number of viewpoints are potentially important. These include the impact on the health status and well-being of patients and of family or friends whose health or social well-being may be affected by providing a joint replacement. In addition, the provision of a joint replacement may have a less direct impact on the health and social well-being of health and social care providers or society in general. This may include feelings of satisfaction or well-being that care is provided to those in poor health, or distress over the impact of any adverse consequences of care (termed as externalities). Finally, joint replacement surgery may have a value to the economy of patients or carers who are able to participate in activities that result in the provision of additional goods or services (termed as indirect costs or benefits).

Whose valuations should be used to derive a summary measure of outcome will depend in part on the decision to be taken. If the decision is whether joint replacement surgery should be available to groups of patients or in a community, then the values should reflect a societal perspective. In this case, utility or monetary values of preferences for health states should be derived from a representative sample of the overall society or community in which the decision to provide joint replacement or care for hip or knee pain is to be taken. This will include a proportion of patients, family or health care professionals concerned with the management of hip or knee pain as well as those who are not directly involved. However, if the decision is whether a specific patient should receive joint replacement surgery then a more limited perspective is appropriate. This would include the patient, their family/friends whose health and social well-being are directly affected and the health professionals responsible for providing care to that patient.

4.6
Who Should Receive Joint Replacement Surgery?

Economic evaluations do not currently incorporate distributional concerns [7]. In economic evaluation, measures of the value of health gain are aggregated to provide a population or societal estimate of value. A key assumption underlying the aggregation is that the social value of a unit of health gain is equal between individuals and across all population groups and that the value is constant over time. In addition, economic evaluation favours those with the greatest capacity to benefit, such as patients more severely affected by osteoarthritis. Using this method of evaluation may systematically discriminate to the advantage of certain groups against others. Inequalities in health between individuals and/or groups of individuals may increase as a result of seeking to maximise health gain.

It has been argued that if measures of health gain such as QALYs represent close approximation of utilities they will incorporate a measure of value for the distribution of health and social well-being and support the maximisation of health gain [7, 8]. However, concern for others' well-being and concepts of justice mean that there are societal preferences for the distribution of that health gain. These differences in valuations may be due to preferences for equity in the distribution of life, life years gained, quality adjusted life expectancy or "just desserts". The latter may be based on a sense of individuals taking some responsibility for engaging in health-promoting behaviour or that individuals who for whatever reason are already disadvantaged should not be made worse off. For example, recent research indicates that the value of health gain varies by patient characteristics such as age and severity of illness prior to care rather than quantity of health or health gain alone [9, 10].

In the case of joint replacement, current utilisation data and predictors of outcome for indicate that decision makers may value equal health gains differently between eligible population groups. Hospital statistics for England and Wales show wide regional variations in operative rates, implying geographical inequalities in access, and American data suggest the elderly, the obese and blacks, are less likely to get a total joint replacement than middle-aged, middle class whites [1]. Some reports also suggest that there is a large unmet need, particularly for knee replacements [1]. This appears to contradict the principle of equal access to or equal treatment of equals, where the determinant is equal need (horizontal equity). However, it could be consistent with horizontal equity if the definition of need includes socio-demographic or economic characteristics as well as the more traditional clinical, functional and disease severity measures. Alternatively it could be consistent with an equal distribution of health or health gain across population groups and/or generations (vertical equity), which would require unequal treatment of unequals.

A recent review suggests that to take distributional concerns into account both individual and societal utilities for health care should be reflected more fully in economic evaluations [1]. It is possible to incorporate concern for equality into cost-effectiveness analysis by using equity weights that represent values for preferences for the distribution of gains in health and social well-being. The greater the equity weight the more society is willing to sacrifice a unit of health gain in pursuit of fairness.

4.7
Summary

In summary, the economics perspective indicates that decisions about whether joint replacement surgery should be available for a population or used for an individual will require evidence about the relative costs and outcomes to the society in which the decisions are taken. This will include those sectors and groups that are responsible for the provision or funding of time, staff, equipment and facilities used as inputs to produce care and those whose health and social well-being is affected by the provision and outcomes of care. Outcomes should include the direct impact on health status and well-being of the patients and others, and measurement and valuation of preferences for those outcomes. Ideally, the evidence should also incorporate preferences for the distribution of the costs and outcomes between sectors and groups of individuals.

4

References

1. Dieppe P, Basler H-D, Chard J et al.: Knee replacement surgery for osteoarthritis: effectiveness, practice variations, indications and possible determinants of utilization. Brit J Rheumatol 1999; 38:73–83
2. Belmar CJ, Barth P, Lonner JH, Lotke PA: Total knee arthroplasty in patients 90 years of age and older. J Arthroplasty 1999; 14(8):911–914
3. De Leeuw JM, Villar RN. Obesity and quality of life after primary total knee replacement. Knee 1998; 5(2):119–123
4. Rissanen P, Aro S, Paavolainen P. Hospital- and patient-related characteristics determining length of hospital stay for hip and knee replacements. Int J Technol Assess Health Care 1996; 12(2):325–335
5. Young NL, Cheah D, Waddell JP, Wright JG. Patient characteristics that affect the outcome of total hip arthroplasty: A review. Can J Surg 1998; 41(3):188–195
6. Gold MR, Siegel JE, Russell LB, Weinstein MC. Cost effectiveness in health and medicine. Oxford University Press, New York, 1996
7. Sassi F, Archard L, Le Grand J. Equity and the economic evaluation of healthcare. Health Technol Assess 2001; 5(3):1–138
8. Bryan B, Roberts T, Heginbotham C, McCallum A. QALY maximisation and public preferences: results from a general population survey. Health Econ 2002; 11:679–693
9. Tsuchiya A. Age related preferences and age weighting health benefits. Soc Sci Med 1999; 48:267–276
10. Dolan P. The measurement of individual utility and social welfare. J Health Econ 1998; 17:39–52

The Cost of the Procedure

5

K. Dreinhöfer, D. Ziegler, G. Röderer, D. Dornacher, and H. Reichel

5.1
Introduction

Total hip arthroplasty (THA) has emerged as one of the most successful interventions in orthopaedics. Many long-term follow-up studies have reported clinical success rates, in terms of patient satisfaction, pain reduction, functional improvement and the absence of further surgery, of greater than 90% at minimum 10-year follow-up evaluation [1]. However, primary THA is an expensive procedure whereas financial resources of health care systems are continuously decreasing and demand for primary total hip replacement is increasing. One major reason for increasing demand is a higher life-expectancy of today's western society with more people at advanced ages suffering from osteoarthritis of the hip and femoral neck fractures. Further reasons are improvements in surgical technique, implant material and design as well as different indication criteria leading to changed thresholds for surgery. Differences in health care systems, total expenditure on health care per capita, population age structure and documentation systems are considered to be reasons for international variations in costs for total hip replacement [2].

Orthopaedic surgeons are more and more required to justify costs for primary total hip replacement. In order to do so, a thorough analysis of costs and costeffectiveness is required which ultimately should lead to the development of strategies to increase the latter and decrease the former.

5.2
Costs

Identifying and evaluating costs are important steps in any economic evaluation. Different aspects of costs have to be considered: direct, indirect and intangible costs [3]. Direct medical costs include all costs that are directly related to the intervention, including those

K. Dreinhörfer (✉)
Department of Orthopedics, Ulm University, Oberer Eselsberg 45, 89081, Ulm, Germany
e-mails: karsten.dreinhoefer@uni-ulm.de; dominik.ziegler@uni-ulm.de;
Daniel.dornacher@uni-ulm.de; heiko.reichel@uniklinik-ulm.de

K.E. Dreinhöfer et al. (eds.), *EUROHIP: Health Technology Assessment*
of Hip Arthroplasty in Europe, DOI: 10.1007/978-3-540-74137-4_5, © 2009 EFORT

5

for personnel, supplies and the facility involved in the treatment. The direct procedure-related hospital costs comprise primarily those of implant, anaesthesia and operating room and nursing/hospital room, in addition to pharmacy, laboratory, radiology, physical therapy, surgical, orthopaedic and central supply [4]. Direct overhead costs are derived from overhead departments (administration, housekeeping, food, laundry, etc.). Furthermore, the costs for rehabilitation, follow-up care and treatment of complications including revision surgery have to be taken into account. Direct non-medical costs include costs borne by patients and their families in the course of treatment (e.g. for transportation or lodging). Indirect costs include costs associated with lost productivity, illness or death, usually valued as lost wages or an imputed monetary value of time. For intangible costs, a money value is assigned to reductions in quality of life associated with pain, suffering and grief.

Beside these costs assessed from the perspective of the health care system, there are additional substantial out-of-pocket costs for the patients undergoing THA, e.g. medications, health professional visits, special equipment, alterations to the house and use of community and private services [5].

The vast majority of the orthopaedic economic evaluations published in the past have been cost-identification (cost-of-illness) or cost-minimisation analyses [6]. With this method, only the costs of a given treatment strategy are considered. By definition, a cost-minimisation study assumes that the outcome of the treatments being analysed are the same or similar [7]. The costs included in the analysis vary depending on the perspectives considered in the study.

5.3
Cost of Total Hip Arthroplasty

Cost in THA varies significantly between different countries all over the world, but also within one country.

In 1997, the total charge for THA across the USA was $20,290, with California 56% above average and Pennsylvania 29% below. The average length of stay was 4.94 days and the per diem cost was $4,110 [8].

In a study from the University of Texas Health Science Center at Houston, the total hospital cost for primary THA in 1992 was $13,826 with a 7.1-day average length of stay. The implant represented 34% of the total costs, followed by anaesthesia and the operating room with 25% and the nursing service and hospital room with 19% [4].

Reuben et al. [9] evaluated the costs for primary THA with a knowledge-based hospital account system for the years 1991–1994 in the same centre. The overall inpatient costs were $16,118 for unilateral and $24,067 for simultaneous bilateral primary THA, the implant costs ranged between 28% and 43% of the total hospital costs.

In comparison, cost-to-charge data were used in a study from the Lahey Clinic in Massachusetts for the years 1993–1995. After the introduction of a cost-containment program, the costs for primary THA was $11,104. Average net income (hospital revenue hospital expense) for primary THA was $2,486 [10].

Bozic et al. [11] analysed 491 consecutive patients at the University of California operated on in 2000–2002 based on an administrative database documenting actual resource utilisation. In this retrospective cost-identification analysis, the mean hospital cost was $24,170 for primary total hip replacements and the average length of hospital stay 5.6 days. Costs incurred in the operating room accounted for more than 50% of the total costs.

Antoniou et al. [12] extracted data from hospital accounting systems of 600 patients from three hospitals in the USA in 2000 and found the median total hospital cost at US$12,846 with an average length of stay of 4.2 days. The overhead costs accounted for 38% of the total. In a comparative analysis, the median cost for THA in three hospitals in Canada was US$6,080 with an average length of stay of 7.2 days and an overhead of 31%.

In an earlier study from Canada, Laupacis et al. [13] calculated the average cost of the initial hospitalisation for 60 THA in 1988 as US $7,452, while the outpatient costs during the first year were US$848 (total cost during the first year US$8,300).

There seems to be an increase in cost for THA over the years. However, Barber and Healy [14] demonstrated that, although there was a 46.5% increase in the actual average cost of the THA from 1981 to 1990, this was only a 1.9% increase in inflation-adjusted dollars [14]. The cost for the patient room decreased from 50 to 37% of the total, whereas the cost for the implant increased from 11 to 24% of the total hospital cost. The dollar price for the implant increased by 212% and the inflation-adjusted dollars cost increased by 117%.

Several European studies have also reported in recent years the cost for primary THA in different countries [15–21].

Table 5.1 summarises these studies from North America and Europe by presenting the length of stay, the implant costs and overall hospital costs expressed in US dollars.

Recent studies revealed that almost 80% of the hospital cost for joint replacement procedures was generated in the operating room, nursing units, recovery room and pharmacy during the first 48 h of hospitalisation [22]. Cost incurred in the operating room accounted for more than 50% of the total hospital costs [11].

Implant costs have a major share in the overall cost of the procedure. Metz and Freiberg [23] reported in an international comparative study a large variation in the cost of THA, as much as 700% for identical implants from a single manufacturer. The average costs for cemented components was $1,536 (range $355–8,440), for uncemented $2,674 (range $100–13,122) and $2,114 (range $100–11,117) for hybrid components.

While implant costs account in Europe for 10–20% [17, 18, 21], in the USA, some reports calculate between 30 and 40% [4, 9, 24]. Major differences are also seen in the direct comparison between Canada and the USA with implant prices varying between US$1,695 and US$8,017 [12].

Overhead costs in the USA are elevated compared to Canada. Antoniou et al. [12] calculated US$2,214 (31.1% of the total costs) for Canada and US$5,118 (37.1%) for the USA, reflecting the higher administrative expenses associated with a multipayer insurance system.

Also cost sensitive is the performance of the procedure in a high- versus low-volume centre. Martineau et al. [25] demonstrated that a THA in a low-volume centre was associated with a 60% increase in total costs. While this was not affected by different co-morbidities, the length of stay was also not significantly different.

Table 5.1 Costs for primary total hip arthroplasty in North America and Europe

Author	Year	Country	Length of stay (in days)	Implant cost (in US$)	Implant cost (in % of total cost)	Total costs (US$)
Barber and Healy [14]	1981	USA – Mass			11	8,428
	1990				24	12,348
Meyers et al. [4]	1992	USA – Texas	7.1	4,769	34	13,826
Reuben et al. [9]	1994	USA – Texas	7.1	4,705	29	Unilateral 16,118
			7.6		43	Bilateral 24,067
Lavernia et al. [24]	1987–90	USA – Maryland	12.0	6,800	40	15,503
Mushinski [8]	1997	US charges	4.9			20,290
Iorio et al. [10]	1991	USA – Mass	8.6	3,840	38	10,210
	1993		5.7	3,461	37	9,446
	1995		4.9			11,104
Bozic et al. [11]	2000–02	USA – California	5.6			24,170
Antoniou et al. [12]	2000	USA	4.2	8,017		12,846
Antoniou et al. [12]	2000	Canada	7.2	1,695	28	6,080
Laupacis et al. [13]	1988	Canada	11.4	1,639	22	7,452
Martineau et al. [25]	1998–2001	Canada	6.3	595	14	High volume 4,403
			7.4	1,695	23	Low volume 7,385
Garellick et al. [15]	1985–1989	Sweden	15.0	1,186	11	9,050
Okhuijsen et al. [16]	1990–1993	Netherlands	14.0	943	19	Cemented 5,058
			12.0	2,157	37	Cementless 5,821
Rissanen et al. [17]	1992	Finland	14.2	2,205	21	10,500
Könning [22]	1991–1993	Germany	22.0	1,341	13	Cemented 10,043
				1,738	17	Cementless 10,473
O'Shea et al. [18]	1999	Ireland	16.4	869	8.2	10,516
Marti-Valls et al. [19]	2000	Spain				4,654
Scheerlinck et al. [21]	2001	Belgium	14.4	1,995	16–21	9,500
Schürmann and Müller [20]	2002	Germany	22.0	1,849	19	Real 9,609
			9.4	1,849	30	DRG-adapted 6,230
Schürmann and Müller [20]	2002	Germany	22.0	1,410	14	Cemented 9,965
				2,073	22	Cementless 9,390

5

Another cost-controlling aspect is the decision for unilateral versus bilateral THA. The cost of single-stage bilateral THA is considerably less than that of two-stage bilateral. Lorenze et al. [26] and Reuben et al. [9] showed a 25% cost saving with bilateral simultaneous total hip arthroplasties. These savings were primarily attributed to the length of hospital stay.

Barrack et al. [27] analysed the cost of implanting cemented versus cementless femoral stems. The average cost for a cementless stem was $900 greater than for cemented. However, the total cost for the accessories used to achieve modern cementation technique was over $700. In addition, the operative time for implanting a cemented stem averaged 20 min longer, which resulted in an additional operating time charge of $270 and additional anaesthesia charges of $100. In summary, the cost for implanting a modern cemented stem was more than $180 greater than implanting a corresponding cementless stem. Laupacis et al. [13] reported no cost difference between the cemented and non-cemented implants and Schürmann and Müller [20] even a little saving with non-cemented implants (€9,390 vs €9,965).

When evaluating all these interesting cost-minimisation analyses one should keep in mind that,by identifying all of the costs associated with a particular treatment, they can be used to compare treatments only when there is strong clinical evidence that patient outcomes are the same or similar [7]. If they are not, focussing solely on costs can lead to misleading results by ignoring important differences in outcomes.

5.4
Economic Evaluation

Orthopaedic surgeons make decisions on the care of their patients and also on hospital and health care policy. Knowledge of the economic analyses of surgical practices is necessary in order to advise in matters of policy. If clinicians are to play a lead role in such discussions, they must develop the skills required for clinical economic analysis [28].

The primary goal of health care economic analysis is to identify interventions that produce the greatest health benefit with the resources available. Most health care economic evaluations are used to compare health outcomes with the relative costs of the resources used to achieve those outcomes. The breadth of outcomes considered varies according to the type of economic analysis performed [3].

The basic types of economic analysis are cost-identification, cost-effectiveness, cost-utility, and cost–benefit analyses. Each of these approaches involves the systematic identification and valuation of the relevant costs and consequences of health care interventions [7]. When combined with clinical trials that evaluate efficacy (the extent to which medical interventions achieve improvements in health under ideal circumstances) and effectiveness (the extent to which medical interventions achieve improvements in health in real practice settings) they provide a decision-making framework that can be useful to both clinicians and health care administrators [3].

Cost-identification analysis (CIA) and cost-of-illness analysis (COIA) measure only the costs associated with a given disease or procedure. No consideration is given to the health consequences. The primary objective of a COIA is to calculate the cost of caring for persons with the illness compared with those who are well, and the goal of a CIA is to calculate the cost of a process or a procedure.

5

Cost-effectiveness analysis (CEA) measures health outcomes in physical or natural units, such as life years gained or patients successfully treated.No attempt is made to value the health outcomes that are reported.Therefore, this technique is appropriate when the outcomes of the different procedures being considered are expected to vary but can be expressed in common natural units. It is the most appropriate method of analysis when the goal is to identify the most cost-effective strategy from among a set of options which produce a common health outcome. However, cost-effectiveness analyses are not helpful for choosing between treatments that have different outcomes or for which the outcomes were measured with different techniques [7]. The use of cost-effectiveness (C/E) ratios has been suggested as a method of simplifying the comparison of results of cost-effectiveness analyses. The goal of using a cost-effectiveness ratio is to compare particular interventions in terms of cost per unit of outcome. When two different health care interventions are compared, an incremental cost-effectiveness ratio is calculated as the difference in cost between the two treatments divided by the difference in effectiveness [3].

Cost-benefit analysis (CBA) measures an intervention in monetary terms. It uses all costs, including an estimation of the productive working time gained by the patient under-going the intervention. However, it undervalues those patients who do not work and has so far not been commonly applied to economic evaluation of THA. The advantage of this type of approach is that it allows comparisons of interventions across subspecialties, as all costs and outcomes are valued in the same monetary units.The goal of CBA is to determine whether the value of the benefits produced (in monetary terms) exceed the value of the resources consumed [3].

Cost–utility analysis (CUA) is similar to CEA except that it incorporates a measure of quality of life or survival into the outcome of the procedure. Such studies are based upon estimating the best and worst imaginable state of health. Quality adjustment involves plac-ing a higher value on time spent in good health than on time spent with impaired physical and emotional function. The units, quality-adjusted life- years (QALYs), are derived and allow comparison between different interventions in term of cost per QALY [7]. This type of analysis is particularly useful when alternative treatments produce outcomes of different types or when longer survival is bought at the expense of reduced quality of life [3].

When measuring QALYs, some limitations have to be addressed. Many ethical assump-tions have to be set regarding what defines quality of life, equity and efficiency, and indi-vidual and societal preferences. Furthermore, decisions based on QALYs (by convention) direct care away from older patients or patients who have a poor quality of life because their care would yield few QALYs at a relatively high cost.

5.5
Economic Evaluation in THA

The number of research publications related to economic topics in THA has increased in recent years. However, the methodology used and the quality of these reports varies. In a recent bibliographic search of MEDLINE databases from 1966 to 2002, only 81 studies contained economic data on THA [6].

Most of these were classified as cost-identification or cost-minimisation analyses (58%) considering only direct costs incurring during the initial peri-operative period. In addition, there were 20 cost-effective analyses (25%), 13 cost-utility analyses (16%) and 1 study was classified as CBA. Of these, 89% considered only direct costs and the majority of studies considered only costs appearing during the time in hospital or rehabilitation. Thirteen studies analysed cost over a time period of more than 12 months. Only three studies used actual cost data collected in a prospective manner.

Liang et al. [29] reported the results of a study on cost-effectiveness of total joint arthroplasty for the treatment of osteoarthritis. They concluded that total joint arthroplasty is more cost-effective for patients with a poor pre-operative health-related quality of life and less effective for patients with better preoperative health status.

Rissanen et al. [17] prospectively analysed cost and cost-effectiveness in THA and total knee arthroplasty (TKA). THA-patients gained more in regard to health-related quality of life and the surgeries were more cost effective than TKR-patients, resulting in a positive C/E ratio.

On a more theoretical basis, Faulkner et al. [30] and Fitzpatrick et al. [31] compared the cost-effectiveness of newer total hip designs with that of conventional prosthesis. Based on prosthesis-specific costs of the primary operation, prosthetic survival data, and morbidity and mortality data, and considering basic economic principles such as discounting and sensitivity analysis, the authors estimated the improvements in outcome and revision rates that would have to be achieved by newer prosthetic designs to justify their additional cost compared with that of the standard Charnley cemented prosthesis.

Daellenbach et al. [32] developed an economic model to calculate the gains in longevity that would have to be achieved by performing total hip arthroplasties without cement to justify their additional cost compared with that of performing total hip arthroplasties with cement. The number of years by which cementless prostheses would have to outlast cemented prostheses in order to justify their additional cost ranges from 4 to 17, depending on the age of the patient, the assumed life of the cemented prosthesis and the predicted cost of revision surgery.

Brauer et al. [33] analysed the English-language medical literature published between 1976 and 2001 for orthopaedic-related cost–utility analyses in which outcomes were reported as cost per QALY. They found six cost–utility ratios for comparisons of THA with the alternative of observation only, and all of the ratios are considered to indicate cost-effectiveness (below a threshold value of $50,000 per QALY) by today's standards.

Chang et al. [34] performed a CUA of THA for osteoarthritis of the hip. Their model was based on detailed hospital cost-accounting data, and they considered both short and long-term outcomes to estimate the cost–utility. THA cost-effectiveness ratio increases with age and is higher for men than for women. In the base-case scenario for 60-year-old white women who have functionally significant but not dependent hip osteoarthritis, the model predicts that THA is cost saving because of the high costs of custodial care associated with dependency due to worsening hip osteoarthritis and that the procedure increases quality-adjusted life expectancy (QALE) by about 6.9 years. In the base-case scenario for men aged 85 years and older, the average lifetime cost associated with THA is $9,100 more than non-operative management, with an average increase in QALE of about 2 years. Thus, the THA cost-effectiveness (C/E) ratio for men aged 85 years and older is $4,600 per QALY gained. On the basis of this analysis, THA can be cost-saving for patients with major functional limitations due to osteoarthritis of the hip or, at worst, cost-effective for improving quality-of-life expectancy.

O'Shea et al. [18] calculated the cost of a QALY for males and females undergoing THA in Ireland in 1999. In the age range of 60–69, the cost per QALY was £1,863 and

£1,467 respectively, while in the age range of 70–79, the respective costs were £3,152 and £2,454. Laupacis et al. [13] calculated the cost per QALY in the USA as $20,245 during the first year and $5,991 during the first 3 years. Lavernia et al. [24] demonstrated that, following hip arthroplasty, the costs per QALY in the USA were $11,560 and $6,656, at 1 and 2 years post-operatively, respectively. Health economists consider an intervention costing less than $30,000 per QALY a bargain to society.

Garellick et al. [15] reported on a gained quality of life after THA in 410 Swedish patients after 1 year and during a 5-year period. The cost utility for the first year was $32,680. If the patient died after 4.5 years, the cost utility was $7,262. With 10 years survival of the patient and the prosthesis, the value would be $3,268 without discounting for the rate of inflation.

However, the costs for health care treatment are difficult to assess because, for most diseases, the costs for the natural course of the disease are unknown. A patient with osteoarthritis of the hip who does not have surgery has expenses for analgesics, physiotherapy, help at home and special transportation. If these costs were taken into account, the costs per QALY gained would be even lower.

In general, the cost utility of THA compares favourably with other medical interventions and demonstrates that THA is one of the most cost-effective surgical interventions as shown in Table 5.2.

Such cost-effective league tables, comparing and ranking health care interventions on the basis of their cost-effectiveness or cost-utility, should be interpreted with caution since the data from these tables are often acquired from different sources. In addition, depending on the time and place of origin, there might be variations in price, clinical practise, technology and access to care. There are also ethical considerations lacking in such calculations and comparisons.

5.6
Strategies to Reduce Costs

Rising health care costs have become an issue of enormous importance in the past two decades. Demographic changes and advances in medical technology have outpaced the ability of most societies to pay for them. Since a further increase of the surgical volume is expected, cost containment becomes very important for the society and the health care providers.

Table 5.2 Cost per quality-adjusted life-years (QALY) of competing therapies (Maynard [35])

Therapy	Cost utility (US$, 1990)
Neurosurgical intervention for head injury	405
Pacemaker implantation	1,805
Hip replacement	1,990
Coronary artery bypass graft (left main vessel disease, severe angina)	3,520
Kidney transplantation	7,930
Heart transplantation	13,200
Coronary artery bypass graft (1 vessel disease, moderate angina)	31,710
Hospital hemodialysis	37,000
Neurosurgical intervention for malignant intracranial tumor	181,500

During the 1980s, the hospital cost for total hip arthroplasties was controlled by decreases in the length of stay in the hospital and in the volume of services delivered.

Over the years, duration of hospital length of stay continued to decrease and so did the financial compensation for the procedure itself. In the meantime, 80% of the hospital costs are generated in the first 48 h [36]. Boardman et al. [37] demonstrated that a further reduction of length of stay did not translate into significant decrease of hospital costs since the volume of service rendered was not reduced by the shorter hospitalisation.

Recent attempts to control or further reduce the hospital cost of joint replacement operations are focussed on controlling the unit costs of personnel and hospital supplies and at controlling the cost of the implant [12].

One approach is the implementation of so-called clinical pathways, flowcharts or algorithms for the complete care of a patient with a clinical problem from the time of diagnosis to the achievement of the desired outcome. Although in the meantime many hospitals have implemented these clinical pathways to standardise the process of care, the effectiveness has not been reviewed extensively. Kim et al. [38] analysed 11 articles comparing outcomes of THA for patients who were treated using clinical pathways as opposed to patients treated without these pathways. They concluded that clinical pathways appear successful in reducing costs [median percent reduction 11% (range 8–38%)], and length of stay in the acute care hospital, with no compromise in patient outcomes. However, interpretation of these studies was complicated by substantial methodological limitations, particularly the use of historical controls in 10 of the 11 studies and failure to account for length of stay in rehabilitation facilities.

Another cost-containment strategy at the hospital level is to reduce the number of different types of prosthesis in one hospital by the introduction of a hip implant standardisation program. Healy et al. [39] reported that the implementation of a clinical pathway and such an implant standardisation program did reduce hospital length of stay and hospital cost, but did not adversely affect the short-term outcome of THA after 2 years. In addition, the development of a Single Price/Case Price Purchasing Program allowed for a specific cost reduction of 32% [40].

On the society level, different strategies to tackle the increasing burden of health costs have been developed and discussed. In the United Kingdom and other places where health care rationing is common, it has been suggested to fund health care programmes in the order in which they appear on a cost-effectiveness league table [41].

Other investigators have analysed the costs for medical technology and compared these financial issues to gain improvements in health status.

Phillips [36] stated that many different types of orthopaedic implants have been developed so far. All of them should prove their quality and even more their superiority to existing well-performing implants. A new model should therefore be cheaper in production costs with equivalent or better long-term results, or it might be more expensive if it has better long-term results compared to existing prostheses. In both cases, not only the direct costs but the costs as a whole, including indirect costs, should be considered. Phillips concluded that only the most effective type of prosthesis is worth being implanted: cheap in production and low revision rates [36].

Briggs et al. [42] examined how much more effective a new prostheses must be, in terms of reducing the need for revision operations, in order to justify this increased cost.

Considering that many of the newer implants, especially the cementless ones, cost over £1,000, this represents a 300% increase in price, even allowing for the possible savings in the cost of cement. With this additional cost, it seemed unlikely to him that new implants will ever save money. However, if purchasers are willing to accept an increase in costs as long as additional benefits are generated, new implants with this sort of additional acquisition cost may be justified for use in younger patients (if a reduction in revision rate of the order of 21–27% can be demonstrated).

Baxter and Bevan [43] developed a cost model to give the present value of using each prosthesis. The present value of prosthesis j is dependent upon three components: the costs of the initial prosthesis, hospital costs of the primary procedure, and the sum of expected future costs of revision. Future costs of revision depend on the age of the recipient and the survival of the implant. All future costs are discounted. The model is based on a number of assumptions: prosthesis revision rates are linear where long-term survival data are not known, mortality rates of THA recipients are equal to those of the general population, account is taken in the model of first revision but not re-revisions, and hospital costs are the same for all types of prosthesis and all patients.

The model is in the form of

$$PV_j = C_j + H + \Sigma \left\{ \frac{L_{mi} \cdot P_{jmi} \left(C_j + H + R \right)}{\left(1 + r \right)^i} \right\},$$

where PV_j is present value of using prosthesis j; C_j is cost of prosthesis j; H is hospital costs including separate categories for theatre costs, ward costs, prophylaxis costs, physiotherapy costs; L_{mi} is probability of a person at age m when receiving a hip arthroplasty being alive in year i; P_{jmi} is probability of prosthesis j in person aged m needing to be revised in year i; R is additional costs of a revision - that is, additional hospital costs; and $1/(1 + r)i$ is a discount factor where r is the discount rate, $i = 0$ to 19 is the year of the primary operation.

Based on the above calculations, Baxter and Bevan [43] stated that, compared with survival data of "centres of excellence" and implant cost of a Charnley prosthesis of £370 including cement, a "no revision" implant should cost no more than about £700 to have equivalent total expected costs over 20 years. They concluded that in 70-year-old women, a low price prosthesis is generally less costly than a high price prosthesis, even with a very low revision rate. In 40-year-old women, prostheses with high prices and low revision rates can be less costly over 20 years than low-priced prosthesis with higher failure rates.

These calculations have not taken into consideration the quality of life of patients with different implants and the impact of repeated and early revisions.

5.7
Conclusion

In conclusion, primary THA is commonly seen as a very effective procedure for improving pain, function and quality of life in patients with arthritis of the hip. THA is also considered to be one of the most cost-effective procedures in medicine. However, to provide a more accurate estimate of the overall cost associated with the THA, future studies should attempt to measure the total costs of THA, including indirect costs incurred by the patients (and society) and downstream costs associated with complications or the need for further intervention, such as revision surgery. If a cost–utility table is used as an instrument for allocating health care resources, it is necessary to do the studies at the same time, in the same hospital or at least country, and to use identical outcome and cost-evaluation methods.

Since the demand for THA by an increasing number of patients will grow further, while the health care resources available seem to be limited, different strategies to reduce the costs have been applied and new strategies will be discussed and tried in the future. Cost containment was originally achieved by shortening the length of stay in the hospital and imposing limitations on the choice of implants which surgeon can use. While the former simply transfers cost to the community, the latter is seen by some to be reasonable when considering hip replacements in the elderly, because more than 95% of primary total hip replacements will outlive their recipients. Since this is not taking quality-of-life aspects into consideration at all, future research has to address prosthesis survival as well as quality of life.

Finally, there is an urgent need for improving economic evaluation in orthopaedics in general and in THA in particular by using standardised methods and transparent reporting. However, it must also be emphasised that economic analysis should be used to inform decisions about clinical practice and policy; it should not dictate them [44]. Economic considerations are only one of many factors and value judgments that should be involved in critical decisions regarding treatment options and allocation of valuable health care resources.

References

1. Soderman P, Malchau H, Herberts P (2000) Outcome after total hip arthroplasty: Part I. General health evaluation in relation to definition of failure in the Swedish National Total Hip Arthoplasty register. Acta Orthop Scand 71(4): 354–359
2. Merx H, Dreinhofer K, Schrader P et al. (2003) International variation in hip replacement rates. Ann Rheum Dis 62(3): 222–226
3. Bozic KJ, Rosenberg AG, Huckman RS et al. (2003) Economic evaluation in orthopaedics. J Bone Joint Surg Am 85-A(1): 129–142
4. Meyers SJ, Reuben JD, Cox DD et al. (1996) Inpatient cost of primary total joint arthroplasty. J Arthroplasty 11(3): 281–285
5. March L, Cross M, Tribe K et al. (2002) Cost of joint replacement surgery for osteoarthritis: the patients' perspective. J Rheumatol 29(5): 1006–1014
6. Bozic KJ, Saleh KJ, Rosenberg AG et al. (2004) Economic evaluation in total hip arthroplasty: analysis and review of the literature. J Arthroplasty 19(2): 180–189
7. Robinson R (1993) Economic evaluation and health care. What does it mean? BMJ 307(6905): 670–673
8. Mushinski M (1999) Average charges for hip replacement surgeries: United States, 1997. Stat Bull Metrop Insur Co 80(2): 32–40
9. Reuben JD, Meyers SJ, Cox DD et al. (1998) Cost comparison between bilateral simultaneous, staged, and unilateral total joint arthroplasty. J Arthroplasty 13(2): 172–179
10. Iorio R, Healy WL, Richards JA (1999) Comparison of the hospital cost of primary and revision total hip arthroplasty after cost containment. Orthopedics 22(2): 185–189
11. Bozic KJ, Katz P, Cisternas M et al. (2005) Hospital resource utilization for primary and revision total hip arthroplasty. J Bone Joint Surg Am 87(3): 570–576

5

12. Antoniou J, Martineau PA, Filion KB et al. (2004) In-hospital cost of total hip arthroplasty in Canada and the United States. J Bone Joint Surg Am 86-A(11): 2435–2439
13. Laupacis A, Bourne R, Rorabeck C et al. (1994) Costs of elective total hip arthroplasty during the first year. Cemented versus noncemented. J Arthroplasty 9(5): 481–487
14. Barber TC, Healy WL (1993) The hospital cost of total hip arthroplasty. A comparison between 1981 and 1990. J Bone Joint Surg Am 75(3): 321–325
15. Garellick G, Malchau H, Herberts P et al. (1998) Life expectancy and cost utility after total hip replacement. Clin Orthop 346: 141–151
16. Okhuijsen SY, Dhert WJ, Faro LM et al. (1998) Een raming van de intramurale kosten van plaatsing van een totaleheupprothese. Ned Tijdschr Geneeskd 142(25): 1450–1455
17. Rissanen P, Aro S, Sintonen H et al. (1997) Costs and cost-effectiveness in hip and knee replacements. A prospective study. Int J Technol Assess Health Care 13(4): 575–588
18. O'Shea K, Bale E, Murray P (2002) Cost analysis of primary total hip replacement. Ir Med J 95(6): 177–180
19. Marti-Valls J, Alonso J, Lamarca R et al. (2000) Efectividad y costes de la intervención de prótesis total de cadera en siete hospitales de Cataluña. Med Clin (Barc) 114(Suppl 2): 34–39
20. Schürmann N, Müller RT (2002) Primäre Endoprothetik am Hüft- und Kniegelenk – Vergleich der Ist-Kosten mit den australischen Diagnosis Related Groups (DRG). Z Orthop Ihre Grenzgeb 140(6): 589–594
21. Scheerlinck T, Duquet W, Casteleyn PP (2004) Socioeconomic aspects of total hip arthroplasty. A one-year survey in a Belgian university hospital. Acta Orthop Belg 70(6): 525–533
22. Healy WL, Iorio R, Richards JA et al. (1998) Opportunities for control of hospital costs for total joint arthroplasty after initial cost containment. J Arthroplasty 13(5): 504–507
23. Metz CM, Freiberg AA (1998) An international comparative study of total hip arthroplasty cost and practice patterns. J Arthroplasty 13(3): 296–298
24. Lavernia CJ, Drakeford MK, Tsao AK et al. (1995) Revision and primary hip and knee arthroplasty. A cost analysis. Clin Orthop Relat Res 311: 136–141
25. Martineau P, Filion KB, Huk OL et al. (2005) Primary hip arthroplasty costs are greater in low-volume than in high-volume Canadian hospitals. Clin Orthop Relat Res 437: 152–156
26. Lorenze M, Huo MH, Zatorski LE et al. (1998) A comparison of the cost effectiveness of one-stage versus two-stage bilateral total hip replacement. Orthopedics 21(12): 1249–1252
27. Barrack RL, Castro F, Guinn S (1996) Cost of implanting a cemented versus cementless emoral stem. J Arthroplasty 11(4): 373–376
28. Haentjens P, Annemans L (2003) Health economics and the orthopaedic surgeon. J Bone Joint Surg Br 85(8): 1093–1099
29. Liang MH, Cullen KE, Larson MG et al. (1986) Cost-effectiveness of total joint arthroplasty in osteoarthritis. Arthritis Rheum 29(8): 937–943
30. Faulkner A, Kennedy LG, Baxter K et al. (1998) Effectiveness of hip prostheses in primary total hip replacement: a critical review of evidence and an economic model. Health Technol Assess 2(6): 1–133
31. Fitzpatrick R, Shortall E, Sculpher M et al. (1998) Primary total hip replacement surgery: a systematic review of outcomes and modelling of cost-effectiveness associated with different prostheses. Health Technol Assess 2(20): 1–64
32. Daellenbach HG, Gillespie WJ, Crosbie P et al. (1990) Economic appraisal of new technology in the absence of survival data – the case of total hip replacement. Soc Sci Med 31(12): 1287–1293
33. Brauer CA, Rosen AB, Olchanski NV et al. (2005) Cost-utility analyses in orthopaedic surgery. J Bone Joint Surg Am 87(6): 1253–1259
34. Chang RW, Pellisier JM, Hazen GB (1996) A cost-effectiveness analysis of total hip arthroplasty for osteoarthritis of the hip. JAMA 275(11): 858–865
35. Maynard A (1991) Developing the health care market. Econ J 101: 1277–1286

36. Phillips H (2003) The economics of total hip replacement. European Instructional Course Lectures 6: 154–157
37. Boardman DL, Lieberman JR, Thomas BJ (1997) Impact of declining reimbursement and rising hospital costs on the feasibility of total hip arthroplasty. J Arthroplasty 12(5): 526–534
38. Kim S, Losina E, Solomon DH et al. (2003) Effectiveness of clinical pathways for total knee and total hip arthroplasty: literature review. J Arthroplasty 18(1): 69–74
39. Healy WL, Ayers ME, Iorio R et al. (1998) Impact of a clinical pathway and implant standardization on total hip arthroplasty: a clinical and economic study of short-term patient outcome. J Arthroplasty 13(3): 266–276
40. Healy WL, Iorio R, Lemos MJ et al. (2000) Single price/case price purchasing in orthopaedic surgery: experience at the Lahey Clinic. J Bone Joint Surg Am 82(5): 607–612
41. Mason J, Drummond M, Torrance G (1993) Some guidelines on the use of cost effectiveness league tables. BMJ 306(6877): 570–572
42. Briggs A, Sculpher M, Britton A et al. (1998) The costs and benefits of primary total hip replacement. How likely are new prostheses to be cost-effective? Int J Technol Assess Health Care 14(4): 743–761
43. Baxter K, Bevan G (1999) An economic model to estimate the relative costs over 20 years of different hip prostheses. J Epidemiol Community Health 53(9): 542–547
44. Gold M, (ed.) (1996) Cost-effectiveness in health and medicine. Oxford University Press, New York

Trends in Hip Replacement Rates

6

M. Flören, P. Dieppe, O. Johnell, and K. Dreinhöfer

It has been shown that there is international variation in the rates of total hip replacement (THR), partly depending on differences in prevalence and incidence of osteoarthritis but also in part related to the health care systems, the total expenditure on health per capita, the age structure and different indication criteria. According to that literature review, the implantation rates for primary THR varied at the end of the last decade between 50/100,000 and 125/100,000 inhabitants in most European countries and the USA.

THR is recognized as cost-effective treatment primarily for osteoarthritis of the hip (70–80%) and fractured neck of the femur (10–20%), and allows for reduction of pain, increased mobility and improved quality of life. Excellent long-term results based on improvements in surgical technique, implant material and design have increased the demand for THR. In addition, joint replacement rates are known to be higher in older age groups and, as the society in the Western World ages, an increase in the number of hip replacements is expected.

Increases in THR rates over the 1990s have been reported in Australia, Germany, the Netherlands, Scandinavia, the UK and the USA.

In the Netherlands, the overall incidence for THR is 20% higher than in Sweden. In the period 1986–1997, the numbers of THR increased by 20% in Sweden and by 68% in the Netherlands [1]. Only 3%and 15%, respectively, of this increase could be explained by changes in the size and age-profile of the population. In this study, it was found that in Sweden, but not in The Netherlands, relatively more elderly people were operated on in 1997 than in 1986.

In the USA,the increase in the number of THR was 23% between 1990 and 1996 [2] and in the UK it was 23% between 1991 and 2000 [3]. The number of operations in patients between the ages of 55–64 and 80 years and over rose significantly over this time period. In South Australia, the overall incidence of THR increased 5% per year between 1988 and 1998 [4], and in Germany 10% between 1998 and 2001 [5].

The proportion of primary and revision hip surgery is similar for most of the countries. One in four hip replacement procedures was a revision in Finland [6], while it was one in five in the UK [3], one in six in Denmark [7] and one in seven in Germany [5] and the USA

M. Flören (✉)
Department of Orthopedics, Ulm University, Oberer Eselsberg 45, 89081 Ulm, Germany
e-mails: markus.floeren@uni-ulm.de;karsten.dreinhoefer@uni-ulm.de

K.E. Dreinhöfer et al. (eds.), *EUROHIP: Health Technology Assessment of Hip Arthroplasty in Europe*, DOI: 10.1007/978-3-540-74137-4_6, © 2009 EFORT

47

[8]. In the Swedish Hip Arthroplasty Registry, the revision rate over the last 20 years was 7.5% for cemented and 17.9% for uncemented THR [9].

Rates of hip replacement revision increased quickly in some countries: in the UK, there has been a 154% increase during the last 10 years (incidence 7.8–19.8), with a dramatic increase in the oldest age group by 477% ($n = 300$) for men and 278% for women ($n = 995$) [3]. The THR revision rate in Germany increased by 13.6% over 4 years (2001 total: 23,500, incidence rate 29/100,000) and in the USA by 24% over 10 years (1991: 25,000, and 2000: 31,000) [5].

These results raise the question whether the increased incidence rate of THR indicates an increased incidence of primary hip osteoarthritis and hip fractures. However, no consistent trend of a change in radiographic prevalence of osteoarthritis was seen over four decades in Sweden [10].

If there is no increased incidence in OA the question remains, what factors could influence the future development of hip replacement rates? Most probably changes in demography and thresholds for surgery will have the strongest impact.

Demographic change is a factor that can be used to estimate future rates since those who will need a hip replacement within the next five decades have all been born. According to estimates by the US Bureau of Census (see Table 6.1), there will be a decline of population in half the European countries within the next five decades by 6.7–12.7% due to reduced birth rates. In contrast, in the other countries, the total population will stay unchanged or will increase by higher birth rates or immigration of people, especially in the USA, by 48%. Irrespective of any change of the total population, the proportion of people older than 50 years will increase in all countries by 12–21%. These rises will lead, even in countries with a decline of population, to an increase in the absolute number of elderly people.

As a consequence of the increasing life expectancy, the absolute numbers in the population at risk for disorders with a predilection for the elderly, such as musculoskeletal conditions, will increase. The people affected by osteoarthritis of the hip and the number potentially demanding a THR will increase as will the incidence of fractures and post-traumatic arthritis. Reasons for these latter changes are an age-associated proneness to falls and an increasing incidence for osteoporosis. According to a German study, the projected numbers for fractures will increase by 13% between 1994 and 2010; in the older age class ($\geq$65 years), the estimated increase in incidence will be 73%.

Differences in the gender ratio of the populations undergoing THR is another factor influencing future trends. The age-standardised incidence of THR is in most countries higher in women then men, especially in the age class $\geq$75 years [1, 3, 11]. This gender difference is explained by different rates of osteoarthritis and osteoporosis, more radiological OA in women or they have a higher disease progression. According to some studies, the prevalence of OA is higher in women than men [12, 13], but in others the incidence is similar [10]. Despite higher implantation rates in women, a Canadian study demonstrated the degree of underuse of THR was more than three times higher in women than in men due to a reduced willingness of women to undergo the procedure [14].

A change in risk factors might also increase the need for arthroplasty. One risk factor is body weight. There is a tendency in industrial nations for body weight to be increasing due to limited physical activities and deficiencies in healthy nutrition. Obesity will probably result in more osteoarthritis cases and more demand for joint replacements. Most epidemiologic

Table 6.1   Demographic changes European countries and USA

Country	Year	Total population	Change in population (%)	Proportion >50 years (%)	Change >50 years (%)
Austria	2000	8,113,413		33.0	
	2025	8,189,560	0.94	46.0	13.0
	2050	7,520,950	−7.30	49.5	16.5
Czech Rep.	2000	10,270,128		32.2	
	2025	9,844,275	−4.15	44.3	12.1
	2050	8,540,221	−16.84	52.8	20.6
Germany	2000	82,187,909		35.5	
	2025	80,637,451	−1.89	47.6	12.1
	2050	73,607,121	−10.44	49.3	13.8
Finland	2000	5,168,595		33.9	
	2025	5,251,272	1.60	43.4	9.5
	2050	4,819,615	−6.75	46.3	12.4
France	2000	59,381,628		32.1	
	2025	63,085,101	6.24	41.6	9.5
	2050	61,017,122	2.75	44.8	12.7
Iceland	2000	281,043		25.2	
	2025	337,632	20.14	35.9	10.7
	2050	350,922	24.86	42.9	17.7
Italy	2000	57,719,337		36.3	
	2025	56,234,163	−2.57	49.4	13.1
	2050	50,389,841	−12.70	52.1	15.8
Netherlands	2000	15,907,853		31.0	
	2025	17,539,636	10.26	42.4	11.4
	2050	17,334,090	8.97	44.7	13.7
Norway	2000	4,492,400		31.6	
	2025	4,916,787	9.45	40.8	9.2
	2050	4,966,385	10.55	44.0	12.4
Poland	2000	38,646,023		27.5	
	2025	38,011,410	−1.64	39.4	11.9
	2050	33,779,568	−12.59	49.3	21.8
Spain	2000	40,016,081		33.0	
	2025	39,578,066	−1.09	46.5	13.5
	2050	35,564,293	−11.12	51.3	18.3
Sweden	2000	8,923,569		36.1	
	2025	9,315,507	4.39	42.4	6.3
	2050	9,084,788	1.81	45.0	8.9
Switzerland	2000	7,266,920		32.7	
	2025	7,774,334	6.98	43.8	11.1
	2050	7,296,092	0.40	50.3	17.6
UK	2000	59,522,468		34.6	
	2025	63,818,586	7.22	41.0	6.4
	2050	63,977,435	7.48	45.3	10.7
USA	2000	282,338,631		27.3	
	2025	349,666,199	23.85	35.7	8.4
	2050	420,080,587	48.79	37.1	9.8

Estimated by the US Bureau of Census (30 April 2004)

6

studies have demonstrated a correlation between overweight and knee osteoarthritis. A similar direct correlation for hip osteoarthritis has not been found in all studies; however, body mass index (BMI) might have a positive predictive value for THR [15].

The threshold for surgery might also have changed. Several factors influence the threshold, like referral from primary care, number of trained orthopaedic surgeons, bed and theatre space, economic restrictions, waiting lists and the existence and application of indication criteria for surgery.

In the last decade, changed indication criteria due to improvements in the THR process has led to THR being offered to a wider selection of patients. Only a few countries have agreed guidelines for indications in THR, in most of the others it is the decision of the surgeon.

Previously, many patients were considered too old or too sick for the procedure and a high complication and mortality rate was expected due to their co-morbidities. On the other hand, THR was refused to younger patients due to disappointing long-term results at the beginning of the joint replacement era.

Over the last 10 years, the number of operations carried out for patients below 64 and above 80 years rose significantly in some countries [1, 3, 4]. This shift in age-classes of patients undergoing THR may be caused by improvements in peri-operative medical care, hip joint prosthesis development, operative techniques and increasing surgical experience, including improved surgical precision and cementing techniques. In addition, especially for uncemented devices, an increased prosthetic survival has been reported.

Other important considerations are the referring physicians and the patients. It seems that there is still a large proportion of people in the society that are eligible for THR because of their pain and functional limitation but who have never contacted a specialist [16]. Different reasons might play a role: some patients, but also some general practitioners, might regard osteoarthritis as a normal part of ageing and not as a disease. In some areas, among those people with severe arthritis, no more than 15% were definitely willing to undergo arthroplasty, emphasising the importance of considering both patients' preferences and surgical indications when evaluating need and appropriateness of rates for surgery [17, 18]. However, as patients become better informed and more aware of present treatments and their risks and benefits, they may be less inclined to accept their disability and prefer treatment at an earlier stage of disease. An increasing number of people expect to remain active and pain-free throughout their lives and are more willing to undergo THR - as well as at a younger and at an older age.

Finally, the demand in the population is not always mirrored by the THR incidence. Economic restrictions in the budget for THR, reflected in waiting lists, might limit the access of patients to the appropriate treatment in many countries.

Assuming no further change in the age- and sex-specific arthroplasty rates, the predicted annual number of THRs by the year 2020 will increase by at least one-fourth in Sweden and almost one-half in the Netherlands [1] (28 and 44%, respectively). Based on the same assumption, the THR rates in the UK will increase by the year 2010 by 7% for women and 15% for men; however, assuming that the rates will continue to increase like in the last 10 years, the projected rates will be 17 and 30% higher, respectively, than in 2000. In countries with a younger population and an expected increase of the overall population, these rates are even more pronounced. In the USA, the expected increases in THR rates are 19% by 2010, 31% by 2015, 46% by 2020 and 77% by 2030 [8]. In New Zealand, the expected increase is 38% by 2015 and 83% by 2030 [19].

The incidence of primary THR for osteoarthritis (OA) varies between countries, but is steadily increasing in all of them. In addition, the rates of THR revisions are increasing even faster. We are unable to predict when and if incidences will stabilise, so estimates of future trends are unreliable. Any future projection must take into account these changing incidences, changes in population demographics, and new guidelines by health insurances, and politics that will react on the increasing discrepancy between demands, provisions and financial resources. Forecasts based on current incidences and demographic changes alone are likely to underestimate future numbers of THR.

References

1. Ostendorf M, Johnell O, Malchau H, Dhert WJ, Schrijvers AJ, Verbout AJ. The epidemiology of total hip replacement in The Netherlands and Sweden: present status and future needs. Acta Orthop Scand 2002;73-3:282–286
2. Praemer A, Furner S, Rice DP. Musculoskeletal Conditions in the United States. Rosemont: American Academy of Orthopaedic Surgeons, 1999
3. Dixon T, Shaw M, Ebrahim S, Dieppe P. Trends in hip and knee joint replacement: socioeconomic inequalities and projections of need. Ann Rheum Dis 2004;63-7:825–830
4. Wells VM, Hearn TC, McCaul KA, Anderton SM, Wigg AE, Graves SE. Changing incidence of primary total hip arthroplasty and total knee arthroplasty for primary osteoarthritis. J Arthroplasty 2002;17-3:267–273
5. Gerster B. Operationshäufigkeit in deutschen Krankenhäusern 1998 bis 2001. In: Klauber J, Robra B (eds.) Krankenhaus-Report 2003. Stuttgart, NY: Schattauer, 2003, pp. 373–409
6. Puolakka TJ, Pajamaki KJ, Halonen PJ, Pulkkinen PO, Paavolainen P, Nevalainen JK. The Finnish Arthroplasty Register: report of the hip register. Acta Orthop Scand 2001;72-5:433–441
7. Lucht U. The Danish Hip Arthroplasty Register. Acta Orthop Scand 2000;71-5:433–439
8. American Academy of Orthopaedic Surgeons. Orthopaedic related statistics. http://www.aaos.org/wordhtml/research/stats/stats_3.htm; accessed 27-07-2004
9. Malchau H, Herberts P, Eisler T, Garellick G, Soderman P. The Swedish Total Hip Replacement Register. J Bone Joint Surg Am 2002;84-A Suppl 2:2–20
10. Danielsson L, Lindberg H. Prevalence of coxarthrosis in an urban population during four decades. Clin Orthop 1997-342:106–110
11. Mahomed NN, Barrett JA, Katz JN, Phillips CB, Losina E, Lew RA, Guadagnoli E, Harris WH, Poss R, Baron JA. Rates and outcomes of primary and revision total hip replacement in the United States medicare population. J Bone Joint Surg Am 2003;85-A-1:27–32
12. Odding E, Valkenburg HA, Algra D, Vandenouweland FA, Grobbee DE, Hofman A. Associations of radiological osteoarthritis of the hip and knee with locomotor disability in the Rotterdam Study. Ann Rheum Dis 1998;57-4:203–208
13. van Saase JL, van Romunde LK, Cats A, Vandenbroucke JP, Valkenburg HA. Epidemiology of osteoarthritis: Zoetermeer survey. Comparison of radiological osteoarthritis in a Dutch population with that in 10 other populations. Ann Rheum Dis 1989;48-4:271–280
14. Hawker GA, Wright JG, Coyte PC, Williams JI, Harvey B, Glazier R, Badley EM. Differences between men and women in the rate of use of hip and knee arthroplasty. N Engl J Med 2000;342-14:1016–1022

6

15. Vinciguerra C, Gueguen A, Revel M, Heuleu JN, Amor B, Dougados M. Predictors of the need for total hip replacement in patients with osteoarthritis of the hip. Rev Rhum Engl Ed 1995;62-9:563–570

16. Fear J, Hillman M, Chamberlain MA, Tennant A. Prevalence of hip problems in the population aged 55 years and over: access to specialist care and future demand for hip arthroplasty. Br J Rheumatol 1997;36-1:74–76

17. Hawker GA, Wright JG, Coyte PC, Williams JI, Harvey B, Glazier R, Wilkins A, Badley EM. Determining the need for hip and knee arthroplasty: the role of clinical severity and patients' preferences. Med Care 2001;39-3:206–216

18. Hudak PL, Clark JP, Hawker GA, Coyte PC, Mahomed NN, Kreder HJ, Wright JG. "You're perfect for the procedure! Why don't you want it?" Elderly arthritis patients' unwillingness to consider total joint arthroplasty surgery: a qualitative study. Med Decis Making 2002;22-3:272–278

19. The Ageing of New Zealand. New Zealand Orthopaedic Association, 2003

Part II

Indication for Hip Replacement

Appropriateness: Consensus in the Criteria for Indications

7

7.1
Introduction

Ontario has had a steady increase in the rate of total hip replacements (THRs) over the past 25 years. There are marked variations within Ontario and across Canada in THRs rates [1, 2]. If one projects the rate increase and takes into account the aging of the population, the number of THRs will more than double, from 8,800 procedures in 2001 to an estimated 20,000 in 2016. Even as provision of THRs increased so have the waiting times for procedures. Beyond THRs patients and those on waiting lists, there are residents who have unmet needs for THRs. Addressing these three issues in health policy, demand for services, waiting times and unmet need, hinges on the appropriateness of the procedure [3, 4].

7.2
Appropriateness of Total Hip Replacement

Pain, functional limitation and radiographic evidence of damage to the hip have been the traditional indications for THRs [5–7], but there is little consensus in a clinical definition of appropriateness. Surveys show wide variations in the indications orthopaedic surgeons employ in making decisions. In one survey, most surgeons required severe daily pain, frequent pain at rest and on transfer, and destruction of most of the joint space on radiograph. For some surgeons, younger age, co-morbidity, technical difficulties and lack of patient motivation worked against surgery, whereas desire to be independent and return to work swayed in favour of surgery [8].

Naylor and Williams [9] worked with an expert panel in Ontario to develop consensus criteria for case selection and surgical priority for total joint replacements (TJRSs), based

J. Williams (✉)
Institute for Clinical Evaluative Sciences, 2075 Bayview Avenue, Toronto, ON M4N 3M5, Canada

K.E. Dreinhöfer et al. (eds.), *EUROHIP: Health Technology Assessment of Hip Arthroplasty in Europe*, DOI: 10.1007/978-3-540-74137-4_7, © 2009 EFORT

on the RAND Delphi panel method [10]. The panel developed case scenarios based on the factors of American College of Rheumatology criteria for functional capacity, levels of pain on activity and rest, and chance of 10-year survival of prosthesis. It was assumed the surgeon would consider perioperative risk, threats to limb viability from vascular disease, potential causes of reduced short-term joint survival, and conditions precluding much functional improvement. Convergence of consensus allowed for the development of algorithms, but the levels of convergence were greater for scenarios for case selection than for the scenarios for surgical priority.

The appropriateness criteria were applied to reviews of medical and hospital charts for patients who had their hips or knees replaced in seven hospitals in an area with a high TJRs rate and eight hospitals in an area with a low rate of TJRs. Two rheumatologists and two orthopaedic surgeons completed the reviews, even though half the records did not have information for all the criteria. The rates of inappropriate cases ranged from 4.4 to 15.8% across the hospitals, regardless of region [11].

Quintana and his colleagues [12–14] extended the RAND Delphi panel method to include the factors of diagnosis, age, surgical risk, previous non-surgical treatments, pain, functional limitation and bone quality. In a prospective study, they applied the criteria for appropriateness to patients undergoing THRs in five large public hospitals in Spain over a 1-year period. Complications were assessed 3 months after surgery, and patients reported on pain, functional limitation and general health 1 year after discharge. The indications for surgery were rated as appropriate (59.3%), uncertain (32.4%) or inappropriate (8.3%), and the ratings did not vary significantly by hospital. Nor were the ratings predictive of outcomes. The ratings of inappropriate and uncertain were related more to indications of moderate levels of pain and functional limitations in patients with osteoarthritis than other scenarios.

Delphi panel criteria are best regarded as screening tests for overuse and under use of specific procedures. They are shaped by a complex interplay of evidence, circumstances and the values of the preferences of experts [15]. While they can be used to adjudicate the need acute hospital care and indicate what should not be done, they are not useful for either accounting for large rate variations across hospitals or small areas or reducing them [15].

In 1998, the Ontario Ministry of Health and Long-Term Care agreed to fund the Ontario Joint Replacement Registry, organized by Bourne and his colleagues in collaboration with the Ontario and Canadian Orthopaedic Associations. The primary purposes of the OJRR are to monitor the effectiveness of TJRs prostheses and procedures and to assist the management of hospital waiting times and lists [16]. Concurrently, the Ministry asked the Institute for Clinical Evaluative Sciences to strike a panel to recommend an information strategy for managing waiting lists and monitoring patient outcomes for primary TJRs. Given the limitations of the Rand Delphi method, the consensus group focussed on using the Western Ontario and McMaster Osteoarthritis (WOMAC) Index as the key indication for appropriateness and outcome. The panel recommended that, at point of consultation, the surgeon complete a standard consultation note and patients complete the WOMAC. At the time the surgeon and patient agree to proceed with surgery, the consultation note and WOMAC responses were to be forwarded to the registry [17].

In the absence of benchmarks for WOMAC scores for defining appropriateness, the panel recommended that patients with severe scores, 50 or higher, be scheduled for surgery within 3 months of the consultation visit. For assessing outcomes, the panel recommended that patients complete the WOMAC at admission for surgery and 1 year after surgery. The data would enable researchers to relate changes in pain and function while on the waiting list and to estimate the impact of severity at consultation on changes in scores while waiting and outcomes [17].

The OJRR project team is working with the recommendations of the panel. Strategies for managing the waiting lists in participating hospitals have yet to be devised. It will take time for the potential of the OJRR to be realized.

7.3
Waiting Lists: Urgency and Appropriateness of Times to Surgery

About half of OECD countries with publically funded hospitals have long waiting lists and elective acute procedures tend to be rationed [18, 19]. This is particularly true for TJRs. At the same time, evidence suggests that waiting times are unrelated to the burden of pain and disability of the patients at the time they elect to have surgery [12, 20–22]. There is consensus that benefits are related to severity of burden and that burden increases with waiting time. However, there is a lack of definitive evidence showing that outcomes are related to waiting times. There are two observational studies that suggest that short waiting times improve outcomes, but they are not conclusive [23, 24] and nor are they definitive.

The New Zealand priority rating project was the first national effort for ordering the queue for surgery and providing funds to increase services. Priority criteria were developed for cataract extraction, coronary artery bypass surgery, hip and knee replacement, cholecystectomy, and tympanostomy tubes for otitis media with effusion. Panels of experts were formed for each elective procedure to develop criteria for identifying the types of patients who would and would not receive surgical services under various levels of funding and for assessing the relative priority of patients in the queues. The criteria were also to ensure consistency and transparency in the provision in surgical services across the health regions of New Zealand [25].

The panels used a two-step Delphi method to identify factors for case selection and the assignment of priority scores to patients. For TJRs, the priority criteria and relative scores (out of 100 points) were pain (degree, occurrence and time walked) –40 points; functional activity –20 points; movement and deformity –20 points, and other factors (multiple joint involvement and ability to work/give care to dependents / live independently) –10 points [25]. There is some evidence that this priority project has resulted in some reductions in waiting times in New Zealand [18, 26].

The Canadian government funded the Western Canada Waiting List Project to develop reliable, valid, practical and clinical transparent measures of priority for five services; cataract surgery, general surgery, hip and knee replacement, MRI and children's mental health [27]. The work was based in part on the results of the New Zealand priority rating project [28]. The panel developed a priority tool with seven items; pain on motion, pain at rest, ability to walk, other functional limitations, abnormal findings, and abilities to work, give care to dependents and/or live independently [29]. In substance and in scoring, it resembles the tool developed in New Zealand. Orthopaedic surgeons completed the form for about 400 patients, and the scores were compared to surgeons' ratings of urgency on a visual analog score and their estimates of maximum acceptable waiting times for the patients [29]. The correlations of among item scores and of priority scores with urgency and maximum acceptable waiting times were deemed sufficient to indicate reliability and validity of the tool [30].

Provinces in Canada have different strategies for managing waiting lists, so the implementation and use of the priority tool is anything but certain. Alberta, British Columbia, Manitoba, Quebec and Saskatchewan have individually developed web-based waiting lists for a number of procedures, including THRs. THRs are elective procedures, and none of the provinces has introduced priority or urgency ratings of patients when they are entered onto the waiting lists.

Reforming the management of waiting lists and waiting times in publicly funded hospital services is designed to make waiting times manageable, not optimal. As in New Zealand, resources and incentives are required for hospital and surgeons to work together to manage waiting lists and reduce waiting times [18]. In Canada, as in other countries, the question becomes: what policy options are there when the services do not meet the demands of patients on waiting lists?

Guaranteed waiting times have been proposed in the Alberta [31] and Senate [32] commissioned reports on health care reform. They recommended that patients waiting for elective procedures should have guaranteed waiting times. Should a patient have to wait beyond a guaranteed time, she or he would be free to have the procedure performed elsewhere at public expense.

Under the Canada Health Act of 1984, all "medically necessary" services are covered under publicly funded health services. Costs of private health care or billing for services beyond the approved schedules for payment are not permissible in our public health system. Both the Alberta and Senate reports called for the introduction of privately funded services to meet the growing demand for elective procedures. Improving the health care system is the top priority for Canadians, and the introduction of a private health sector is a key issue in the debate.

OECD studies report that guaranteed waiting times have been tried and abandoned in England and Sweden [18, 19]. Initial attempts to managing guaranteed waiting times included the minimum scores required for entry on a waiting list, thereby controlling the numbers eligible for the guarantee. The median waiting times did not decrease, and some physicians provided to patients according to guaranteed waiting times rather than clinical priorities.

Canada has a Charter of Rights, which is part of the constitution. Dr. Jacques Chaouilli, a family physician, and George Zeliotis brought a case to the Quebec courts. They argued that Zeliotis had to wait months in pain for a hip replacement, the public system denied him the right purchase care, and this was a denial of a basic right to medically necessary services. The Quebec courts ruled against the petitioners, and now the case is before the Supreme Court of Canada [33]. Provincial governments, private interest groups and politicians are making presentations to Supreme Courts on the issues involved. Timely care to avoid burden of disability is becoming a basic human right.

7.4
Appropriateness and Unmet Need: In the Community and in the Queue

Inequities in need exist in the community among patients in the queue and persons with hip disease who have not been assessed by their primary care physicians. There may be more persons disabled by pain and disability from damaged hips who have not been assessed for surgery than persons in the queue [21, 34–36].

Hawker and her colleagues are studying a cohort of persons 55 years of age and older in two areas in Ontario, one area with high TJRs rates and one area with low TJRs rates [34–36]. After excluding persons who had surgery or who are on waiting lists, 4.5% of older women and 2.1% of older men were deemed appropriate candidates for arthroplasty, based on WOMAC scores of patients having TJRs in Ontario [36]. When presented with a statement of the risks and benefits of surgery, about one in nine of those persons were willing to consider TJRs. The other eight were willing to live with the burden of osteoarthritis.

In a qualitative study, 17 potential candidates for TJRs gave three reasons for deferring a decision [37]. Some participants viewed osteoarthritis as a normal part of aging, not as a disease. Many of them believed that their pain and disability had to be worse before they would be considered as candidates. Lastly, some participants believed that their physicians would advise them as to when they should consider surgery and be referred to an orthopaedic surgeon. The findings suggest that physicians should reconsider how patients view their osteoarthritis and their disabilities and how the benefits of surgery might best be addressed.

7.5
Conclusion

THR is a medically necessary procedure for managing osteoarthritis and other diseases of the hip. There is consensus on criteria that should be used to evaluate the appropriateness for surgery, and on the clinical presentations, pain, disability and other factors of importance to the patient. There is less agreement on how the criteria should be articulated into a measure. Current measures and tools serve to define cases of minor and major severity, but they work less well to sort through the uncertainties associated with moderate pain and disability. Nonetheless, by whatever set of criteria employed, there is consensus that most hip patients are appropriate for surgery.

There is little consensus on whether outcomes of surgery improve with shorter waiting times. Measures of priority or urgency are based on assumptions rather than data, hence it is difficult to work them into systems for managing waiting lists and waiting times.

Given the unmet need, if not the growing demand for THRs, there is the question as to whether primary care physicians and orthopaedic surgeons should be proactive in discussing patient conditions with respect to appropriateness for, and the benefits of, surgery. The goals would be to reduce unmet need and the inequalities in access to services.

7

The problem of waiting lists is greater in countries with publicly funded services than in countries with a mix of public and private services. Countries such as Canada will either have to find ways to provide necessary services within acceptable waiting times or be faced with prospect of organising services to guarantee the basic rights of its citizens.

References

1. Williams JI. publication in press
2. Canadian Joint Replacement Registry 2003 Report. Total hip and total knee replacements in Canada. Ottawa: Canadian Institute for Health Information, 2003
3. Shortt SED, Shaw RA. Equity in Canadian health care: does socioeconomic status affect waiting times for elective surgery? Canadian Medical Association Journal 2003;168(4):413–416
4. Sanmartin C, Shortt SED, Barer ML, Sheps S, Lewis S, McDonald PW. Waiting for medical services in Canada: lots of heat, but little light. Canadian Medical Association Journal 2000;162(9):1305–1310
5. Quinet RJ, Winters GE. Total joint replacement of the hip and knee. Medical Clinics of North America 1992;76:1235
6. Thompson RC, Gustilo R, Biebel JH, et al. Total hip replacement practice guidelines and recommendations. Minneapolis, MN: Minnesota Clinical Comparison and Assessment Project, Council of Hospital Corporations, 1991
7. Total Hip Replacement. NIH Consensus Statement Online 1994 September 12–14;12(5):1–31
8. Mancuso CA, Ranawat CS, JM Esdaile JM, Johanson NA, Charlson ME. Indications for total hip and total knee arthroplasties: results of orthopaedic surveys. Journal of Arthroplasty 1996;11:34–46
9. Naylor CD, Williams JI. Ontario panel on hip and knee arthroplasty. Primary hip and knee replacement surgery: Ontario criteria for case selection and surgical priority. Quality in Health Care 1996;5:20–30
10. Brook RH, Chassin MR, Fink A, Solomon DH, Kosecoff J, Park RE. A method for the detailed assessment of the appropriateness of medical technologies. International Journal of Technological Assessment in Health Care 1986;2:53–63
11. Van Walraven C, Paterson JM, Kapral M, Chan B, Bell M, Hawker G, Gollish J, Schatzker J, Williams JI, Naylor CD. Appropriateness of primary total hip and knee replacements in regions of Ontario with high and low utilization rates. Canadian Medical Association Journal 1996;155(6):697–706
12. Quintana JM, Arostegui I, Azkarate J, Goenaga JI, Guisasola I, Alfageme A, Diego A. Evaluation by explicit criteria of the use of total hip joint replacement. Rheumatology 2000;39(11):1234–1241
13. Quintana JM, Arostegui I, Azkarate J, Goenaga JI, Tobio R, Aranburu JM, Goikoetxea B. Use of explicit criteria for total hip joint replacement fixation techniques. Health Policy 2002;60(1):1–16
14. Quintana JM, Azkarate J, Goenaga JI, Arostegui I, Beldarrain, Villar JM. Evaluation of the appropriateness of hip joint replacement techniques. International Journal of Technology Assessment in Health Care 2000;16(1):165–177
15. Naylor CD. What is appropriate care? New England Journal of Medicine 1998;338(26):1918–1920
16. Ontario Joint Replacement Registry.http://ojrr.ca/ojrr/public/
17. Blackstein-Hirsch P, Golish JD, Hawker G, Kreder H, Mahomed N, Williams JI. Information strategy: urgency rating, waiting list management, and patient outcomes monitoring for primary hip/knee joint replacement. Toronto: Institute for Clinical Evaluative Sciences, 2000

18. Siciliani L, Hurst J. Tackling excessive waiting times for elective surgery: a comparison of policies in twelve OECD countries. OECD Health Working Papers No. 6. Paris: OECD, 2003

19. Hurst J, Siciliani L. Explaining waiting times for variations for elective surgery across OECD countries. OECD Health Working Papers No. 7. Paris: OECD, 2003

20. Williams JI, Llewellyn-Thomas H, Arshinoff R, Young N, Naylor CD. Ontario Hip and Knee Replacement Project Team. The burden of waiting for hip and knee replacements in Ontario. Journal of Evaluation in Clinical Practice 1997;3:59–68

21. Derrett S, Paul C, Morris JM. Waiting for elective surgery: effects on health-related quality of life. International Journal for Quality in Health Care 1999;11:47–57

22. Fitzpatrick R, Norquist JM, Reeves BC, Morris RW, Murray DW, Gregg PJ. Equity and need when waiting for total hip replacement surgery. Journal of Evaluation in Clinical Practice 2004;10:3–9

23. Fortin PR, Penrod J, Clarke A, St-Pierre Y, Joseph L, Belisle P. Timing of total joint replacement affects clinical outcomes among patients with osteoarthritis of the hip and knee. Arthritis and Rheumatism 2002;46:3327–3330

24. Mahon JL, Bourne RB, Rorabeck CH, Feeney DH, Stitt L, Webster-Bogaert S. Health-related quality of life and mobility of patients awaiting elective total hip arthroplasty: a prospective study. Canadian Medical Association Journal 2002;167(10):1115–1121

25. Hadorn DC, Holmes A. The New Zealand priority criteria project. Part I: Overview. British Medical Journal 1997;314:131–134

26. Gauld R, Derrett S. Solving the surgical waiting list problem? New Zealand's 'booking system'. International Journal of Health Planning and Management 2000;15:259–272

27. Noseworthy TW, McGurran JJ, Hadorn DC. Steering Committee of the Western Canada Waiting List Project. Waiting for scheduled services in Canada: development of priority-setting scoring systems. Journal of Evaluation in Clinical Practice 2003;9:23–31

28. Hadorn DC. Steering Committee of the Western Canada Waiting List Project. Setting priorities on waiting lists: point count systems as linear models. Journal of Health Services Research and Policy 2003;8:48–54

29. Arnett G, Hadorn DC. Steering Committee of the Western Canada Waiting List Project. Developing priority criteria for hip and knee replacement: results from the Western Canada Waiting List Project. Canadian Journal of Surgery 2003;60:290–295

30. Conner-Spady BL, Arnett G, McGurran JJ, Noseworthy TW. Steering Committee of the Western Canada Waiting List Project. Prioritization of patients scheduled waiting lists: validation of a scoring system for hip and knee arthroplasty. Canadian Journal of Surgery 2004;47:39–46

31. Mazankowski D. A framework for reform: report of the Premier's Advisory Council on Health.www.premiersadvisory.com/reform.html

32. Standing Senate Committee on Social Affairs, Science and Technology. The Health of Canadians – The Federal Role, Volume Six: Recommendations for Reform. Ottawa: Senate of Canada, 2002

33. Walkom T. Senators joint court challenge of medicare. Toronto Star, February 12, 2004

34. Hawker GA, Wright JG, Coyte PC, Williams JI, Harvey B, Glazier R, Wilkins A, Badley EM. Determining the need for hip and knee arthroplasty: the role of clinical severity and patients' preferences. Medical Care 2001;39(3):206–216

35. Hawker GA, Wright JG, Coyte PC, Williams JI, Harvey B, Glazier R, Badley EM. Differences between men and women in the rate of use of hip and knee arthroplasty. New England Journal of Medicine 2000;342(14):1016–1022

36. Hawker GA, Wright JG, Glazier RH, Coyte PC, Harvey B, Wilkins A, Badley EM. The effect of education and income on need and willingness to undergo total joint arthroplasty. Arthritis and Rheumatism 2002;46(12):3331–3339

37. Hudak PL, Clark JP, Hawker GA, Coyte PC, Mahomed NN, Kreder HJ, Wright JG. "You're perfect for the procedure! Why don't you want it?" Elderly arthritis patients' unwillingness to consider total joint arthroplasty surgery: a qualitative study. Medical Decision Making 2002;22(2):272–278

Radiographic Assessment of Indications for Total Hip Replacement

8

M. Dougados

8.1
Is There Any Role of Radiological Assessment for Considering Total Hip Replacement?

There are several possibilities permitting to answer this question:

1. Check the available set of recommendations for considering total articular arthroplasty
2. Evaluate the longitudinal studies of hip disease permitting to check the weight of the radiological aspect of the disease in the decision for performing total hip arthroplasty

8.1.1
Sets of Criteria for Total Hip Replacement

To our knowledge, five sets of criteria for total hip replacement have been proposed [1–5].

The National Institute of Health has suggested that total hip replacement be considered in patients with radiographic evidence of joint damage, persistent pain and disability interfering with daily activities, and should not be recommended for patients at high risk of infection or those in poor general health [5]. This provides a very general statement rather than a set of criteria; this statement is not referring at all to any radiological aspect of the disease.

Hawker et al. [2] defined potential candidates for total hip replacement as patients with a summed Western Ontario MacMaster University (WOMAC) OA Index score ≥39, clinical and radiographic evidence of arthritis, and no absolute contra-indication to total hip replacement. The estimate of potential need was then adjusted for willingness. The advantage of this set of criteria is that it is data-driven. The cut-off WOMAC score of 39 represents the 25th percentile of scores for patients undergoing hip or knee arthroplasty in Ontario. With regard to the potential utilisation of total hip replacement as an outcome measure, the

M. Dougados
René Descartes University, Assistance Publique – Hôpitaux de Paris, Cochin Hospital,
27 rue du Faubourg, Saint Jacques, 75014 Paris, France
e-mail: m.doug@cch.ap-hop-paris.fr

K.E. Dreinhöfer et al. (eds.), *EUROHIP: Health Technology Assessment*
of Hip Arthroplasty in Europe, DOI: 10.1007/978-3-540-74137-4_8, © 2009 EFORT

8

drawbacks of these criteria are that they do not take into account either the structural severity of the disease or variability in antecedent pharmacological and non-pharmacological
therapy, and also that they are sensitive to fluctuations in disease activity over time,
co-morbidity and the patient's willingness to undergo total hip replacement. They do not
indicate which patients need total hip replacement, but in which patients total hip replacement is performed in Ontario, Canada.

The Lequesne index [3] is currently used as an outcome measure in clinical trials, but
was designed as an index for patients with OA who were under consideration for total hip
replacement. Based on the clinical experience of the author, it is reasonable to consider
total hip replacement in patients who have a score >10–12 (possible range = 0–24). This
index does not take into account the structural severity of the disease or therapeutic variables. It is sensitive to fluctuations in disease activity over time, and the cut-off value is
imprecise and intuitive. However, the author has recently re-examined the cut-off value
and now recommends a data-driven score of 12 as a cut-off for total hip replacement [6].
This threshold predicted with the best accuracy the occurrence of total hip replacement in
patients included in the ECHODIAH study [7].

The New Zealand criteria [1] are based on the sum of a set of scores for a variety of
clinical factors, including pain, functional impairment, range of motion, deformity and
other features, such as the impact of the disease on life style. They do not take into account
the structural severity of OA or therapeutic variables, but are sensitive to fluctuations in
disease activity over time. To our knowledge, no cut-off value has been validated. However,
recently, a cross-sectional epidemiological study aimed at evaluating how many people in
England are justifying a primary knee replacement surgery used the value of 55 above
which such intervention might be justified [8].

The composite index proposed by our group from Cochin Hospital in Paris is based on
symptomatic severity (the patient's assessment of disease activity and the Lequesne Index) and
structural severity, and on the response to prior pharmacological and non-pharmacological
therapies [4]. This provides a data-driven set of criteria for total hip replacement established
by the evaluation of a large cohort of patients who were followed over 3 years.

Two indices were proposed, which differed on the basis of how the symptomatic and
therapeutical variables were collected. The first index, which used a collection of variables
obtained at a single point in time (see Table 8.1), is easier to use than the second index, which
requires two evaluations at a 3-month interval. The advantage of the second index, however,
is that it is theoretically less sensitive to fluctuations in disease severity over time. The
Cochin's indices offer several advantages: they are easy to collect, and the domains and tools
used for evaluation are valid, reliable and have been recommended by several societies,
including Outcome Measures in Rheumatology (OMERACT) and the Osteoarthritis Research
Society International (OARSI) [9, 10]. They include numerous parameters associated with
total hip arthroplasty, such as disability, effects on lifestyle, concomitant treatment and structural severity. Their disadvantage is that they do not indicate which patients require total hip
arthroplasty but, rather, in which patients total hip arthroplasty is performed in France.

In summary, sets of criteria for considering total hip replacement are usually referring
only to the presence of radiological evidence of osteoarthritis but not to the fact that such
a radiological parameter should demonstrate an advanced disease. In fact, when performing multivariate analysis on the characteristics of the patients who are undergoing total hip

Table 8.1 Proposed composite index for considering total arthroplasty in hip osteoarthritis (adapted from [4])

Characteristic	Grades of the variables	Score[a]
Joint space width on the last available X-ray	>2 mm	0
	≤2 mm and >1 mm	20
	≤1 mm	35
Patient's overall assessment (none = 0, mild = 1, moderate = 2, severe = 3, very severe = 4)	≤2	0
	>2	15
Lequesne's index	≤12	0
	>12	25
NSAIDs intake during the 3 months preceding the visit	≤1 day/2	0
	>1 day/2	15
Analgesic intake during the 3 months preceding the visit	≤1 day/week	0
	>1 day/week	10

[a] A total score (sum of the five sub-scores) below 40 was rarely observed in patients undergoing surgery

replacement, the results clearly show that the radiological appearance (level of joint space narrowing) is an important factor in explaining the surgery.

8.1.2
Longitudinal Study

We took the opportunity to get prospective longitudinal (radiological symptomatic and therapeutical information of a large cohort of patients (>500), followed over 3 years to evaluate in a multivariate analysis the differences existing between those patients who had to undergo surgery ($n = 106$) and those who had not ($n = 400$). When focussing the analysis on the radiological severity (defined by the joint space narrowing), we evaluated not only the absolute joint space width value observed either at the end of the 3-year follow-up period (for those patients who did not have to undergo surgery) or just before surgery (for those who had to undergo surgery), but also in the changes in joint space width evaluated in millimeter per year between the beginning of the study and either the time of surgery or the end of the 3-year follow-up period [11]. The results summarised in Table 8.2 clearly showed that patients who underwent surgery had not only a more advanced disease but also a more rapid progression, suggesting that such an aspect (rapidly progressive disease) is one of the important aspects to take into account when considering surgery [12, 13].

In this case (rapidly structural progression disease), we also showed that the symptomatic severity of the disease was also increased [11]. This rapid symptomatic and structural deterioration does not give patients and doctors more time to adjust and to accept increasing severity [14], probably explaining the high rate of surgical intervention in such cases.

This has been confirmed in the same cohort of patients we subsequently continued to follow-up to 5 years. In this study, we evaluated the changes in joint space width during the first 2 years and thereafter the requirement to total hip replacement during the next 3 years of follow-up of these patients. We found a close correlation between the changes in the joint

8

Table 8.2 Radiological severity (joint space width) in patients undergoing or not hip arthroplasty in a 3 year longitudinal study of a cohort of 506 hip osteoarthritic patients (adapted from [11])

Radiological characteristic joint space width	Total hip replacement during the study	
	Yes $n = 106$	No $n = 400$
Last value (mm)	0.8 ± 0.9	1.8 ± 1.0
Changes during the study:		
• mm/year	-1.0 ± 1.4	-0.2 ± 0.5
• Change > 0.5 mm	67%	35%

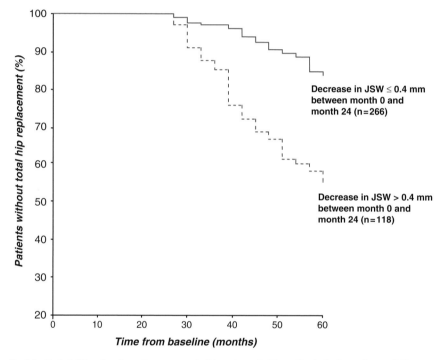

Fig. 8.1 Probability of undergoing surgery in hip osteoarthritic patients during a 3-year follow-up period with regard to a previous 2 years radiological change in joint narrowing

space width after 2 years of follow-up and the requirement to surgery between year 2 and year 5. Using a ROC curve analysis, it was possible to define, as a change of at least 0.4 mm, the optimal cut-off permitting the prediction of such surgery, since the probability to undergo surgery in the group of 118 patients who had a radiological deterioration was 68% compared to 33% in the other group of 266 patients who did not have a radiological deterioration during the first 2 years of follow-up [15]. These results are illustrated in Fig. 8.1.

In summary, despite the fact that some recommendations are not referring at all to the radiological aspects of the disease, it seems that, in practice, the radiological appearance and in particular its severity is considered as important at least for the general practitioners and the rheumatologists.

8.2
Which Are the Different Radiological Aspects Which Might Be of Interest when Considering Total Articular Replacement?

8.2.1
The Confirmation of a Hip Arthropathy and in Particular Osteoarthritis

It is usually admitted that, in case of osteoarthritis, all the different cardinal radiological signs must be observed:

- Joint space narrowing
- Osteophytes
- Subchondral bone sclerosis
- Subchondral cysts

8.2.2
The Diagnosis of an "Advanced" Disease

An "advanced" disease is usually defined by an important joint space narrowing. Clearly, there is no well-accepted definition of "important joint space narrowing". In our longitudinal database, a joint space width below 1 mm at the narrowest point was found to highly predict a subsequent requirement to surgery

We have previously discussed the question of the "rapidly progressive hip osteoarthritis" which might result, in daily practice, to prescribe iterative pelvic X-rays in case of a persistent painful hip osteoarthritis, usually observed in the elderly [12, 13].

8.2.3
The Aetiology of Hip Osteoarthritis

As a rheumatologist, the author will not detail the consequences concerning the surgical procedure based on a specific osteoarthritis aetiology such as important coxa vara or coxa valga.

Moreover, hip OA occurring in the course of a DISH (diffuse idiopathic skeletal hyperostosis) might be important to consider since the postoperative ossification might be more frequent in such a condition [16].

8

8.3
In Conclusion

Radiological assessment of osteoarthritis is of great importance when considering hip arthroplasty. Besides the implications concerning the surgical procedure, it is the opinion of the author that such assessment has to be taken into account in the decision to consider hip arthroplasty.

References

1. Hadorn HC, Holmes AC. Education and debate: the New Zealand priority criteria project, part I: overview. Br Med J 1997;314:131–134
2. Hawker GA, Wright JG, Coyte PC, Williams JI, Harvey B, et al. Differences between men and women in the rate of use of hip and knee arthroplasty. N Engl J Med 2000;342:1016–1022
3. Lequesne M. The algofunctional indices for hip and knee osteoarthritis. J Rheumatol 1997;24:779–781
4. Maillefert JF, Gueguen A, Nguyen M, Berdah L, Lequesne M, et al. A composite index for total hip arthroplasty in patients with hip osteoarthritis. J Rheumatol 2002;29:347–352
5. NIH consensus development panel on total hip replacement. JAMA 1995;273:1950–1956
6. Lequesne M, Taccoen A. Clinical and radiographic status of patients in the ECHODIAH study who underwent THA. Pertinence of the pain-function index for operative decision making. Presse Med 2002;31:4518–4519
7. Dougados M, Nguyen M, Berdah L, Mazières B, Vignon E, et al. Evaluation of the structure-modifying effects of diacerein in hip osteoarthritis: ECHODIAH, a three-year, placebo-controlled trial. Arthritis Rheum 2001;44:2539–2547
8. Juin P, Dieppe P, Donovan J, Peters T, Eachus J, et al. Population requirement for primary knee replacement surgery: across-sectional study. Rheumatology 2003;42:516–521
9. Bellamy N, Kirwan J, Boers M, Brooks P, Strand V, et al. Recommendations for a core set of outcome measures for future phase III trials in knee, hip, and hand osteoarthritis. Consensus development at OMERACT III. J Rheumatol 1997;24:799–802
10. Hochberg MC, Altman RD, Brandt KD, Moskowitz RW. Design and conduct of clinical trials in osteoarthritis. Preliminary recommendations from a task force of the osteoarthritis research society. J Rheumatol 1997;24:792–794
11. Dougados M, Gueguen A, Nguyen M, Berdah L, Lequesne M, et al. Requirement for total hip arthroplasty: an outcome measure of hip osteoarthritis? J Rheumatol 1999;26:855–861
12. Lequesne M. Les coxopathies destructrices. Rev Rhum Mal Osteoart 1970;37:711–719
13. Rosenberg ZS, Shankman S, Steiner G et al. Rapid destructive osteoarthritis: clinical, radiographic and pathologic features. Radiology 1992;182:213–216
14. Day RO. Pharmacokinetic and pharmacodynamic aspects of the ideal COX-2 inhibitor: a rheumatologist's perspective. ClinExp Rheumatol 2001;19(suppl 25):S3–S8
15. Maillefert JF, Gueguen A, Nguyen M, Berdah L, M Lequesne, et al. Relevant change in radiological progression in patients with hip osteoarthritis. Part II: Determination using an expert approach. Rheumatology 2002;41:148–152
16. Arlet J, Jacqueline F, Depeyre M, Mazieres B, Gayrard M. La hanche dans l'hyperostose vertébrale. Rev Rhum Mal Osteoart 1978;45:17–26

Patients' Views on Total Joint Replacement in the UK

9

G. Woolhead, C. Sanders, and P. Dieppe

9.1
Introduction

Approximately 70,000 hip and knee procedures are performed in English hospitals each year [1], causing lengthy waiting lists for total joint replacements (TJR) within the National Health Service (NHS). Most patients have to wait for many months for an initial appointment to see an orthopaedic surgeon, and a further 6–18 months before they are put on the TJR waiting list. Some wait for shorter times than others, and a proportion of those referred to NHS surgeons for consideration of joint replacement are not put on the waiting list, being told that surgery is not appropriate for them. These findings imply that choices are being made as to who should have an operation and which cases should be prioritised [2, 3]. There are also concerns about unmet need for treatment of severe arthritis in the UK and underprovision of total knee joint replacements [4, 5]. Recent reviews have highlighted variations in surgical activity at both national [1] and international levels [6], with the US, for example, having much higher rates of total knee replacement (TKR) than the UK. Rates of TJR also vary by age, gender, ethnicity and, socio-economic status [7, 8], despite there being no evidence that such factors affect outcome [7–9].

As part of a programme of research into the provision of TJR surgery in the UK, two qualitative studies investigated the views of recipients (and potential recipients) on their perceived need for TJR, their experiences of seeking and accessing surgery, and their views on priorities for surgery.

9.2
Methodology

The use of qualitative research to provide data that cannot easily be captured in quantitative form has become established in the conduct of health-related research [10, 11]. Such an approach was considered particularly valuable for these two studies because the accept-

G. Woolhead (✉)
Medical Research Council, Health Services Research Collaboration, Dept. of Social Medicine, University of Bristol, Canynge Hall, Whiteladies Road, Bristol, BS8 2PR, UK
e-mails: gillian.woolhead@bristol.ac.uk; P.Dieppe@bristol.ac.uk

K.E. Dreinhöfer et al. (eds.), *EUROHIP: Health Technology Assessment*
of Hip Arthroplasty in Europe, DOI: 10.1007/978-3-540-74137-4_9, © 2009 EFORT

9

ability and desirability of surgery to patients is essential for any assessment of need and provision of TJR. Work based on survey data can provide some insight into patient views, but such an approach is necessarily limited and constrained. Consequently, qualitative interviews were adopted to allow greater flexibility and exploration of patient views in these two studies.

Qualitative research uses non-probability sampling methods, as the aim is to increase the insight into social phenomena, rather than produce statistically generalisable findings. In both studies, the sampling for the in-depth interviews was purposive. This is where the research guides the sampling and data collection procedure. In the first study, CS carried out in-depth interviews with participants in the community who had moderate to high levels of hip/knee pain and disability (according to New Zealand Priority Criteria scores). Forty-six people were invited for in-depth interview, and 27 consented. There were 10 men and 17 women; median age 76 years (range 51–91). In the second study, carried out by G.W., individuals were purposefully selected from the TKR waiting lists. Of the 40 patients approached, 25 gave their consent and in-depth interviews were conducted 3 months before their TKR. There were 14 women and 11 men; median age 68 years (range 40–84).

In both the studies, in-depth interviews were carried out in people's homes with the aid of a checklist, to explore informants' views on patient selection and prioritisation, perceptions of need for joint replacement surgery and their experiences of consultation with health professionals for treatment. All the interviews were transcribed verbatim (except two where detailed notes were made) and analysed inductively using some of the techniques of grounded theory [12]. Thus, the processes of sampling, data collection and analysis were continuous and iterative, in that later interviews built on earlier analysis and allowed the exploration of issues arising. Data were analysed by detailed scrutiny of the transcripts to identify common themes, which were then coded, using the computer software package Atlas.ti. "Negative" or deviant cases were identified and scrutinised carefully. The coding and analysis were discussed regularly at team meetings in order to refine and develop the analytic process.

9.3
Results

In analysing the interview data, it was clear that patients considered the degree of their symptoms and disability important when assessing their needs for treatment. However, beyond this, their assessments of whether or not they needed surgery, and the issue of when such surgery would be appropriate, was dependent on many other considerations. The issue of age was central to patients' perceptions of their need for surgery and the appropriate timing of an operation. Additional factors were also mentioned in their self-assessments of need for surgery such as weight, co-morbidity and personal issues such as caring commitments. Moreover, their self-assessments of the need for and timing of surgery were mediated by their consultations with physicians, who would either confirm or counteract their own views. Here, the capacity for community physicians to act as "gatekeepers" to specialist hospital care was evident, as were the differing priorities between patients and physicians. Further details and illustrations are given below.

9.3.1
Pain and Disability as Indicators of Surgical Need

In both studies, most of the respondents had experienced the pain and disability of arthritis for one or more decades and tended to perceive their symptoms as being inevitable and associated with normal ageing. Consequently, many believed (or had believed in the past) that they could tolerate or endure the pain and disability of OA, and felt that little formal treatment could be offered to them. This pessimism represented a major factor in making them reluctant to seek formal health care:

> "…it doesn't get better and we know there's no cure for it. When you know that there isn't a cure for it that puts a great deal of difference to it. It isn't like when you've got a cold and you know that's gonna pass off and you're gonna get better, but with arthritis it never gets better" (female, age 82)

In G.W.'s study, many stated that they had delayed seeking health care and held a stoical attitude over their own pain and disability. For example, several compared themselves to other people worse off than themselves, leading to some respondents feeling less inclined to complain or ask for help:

> "…I keep out of the doctors, there are worse off than me so I keep out… the only time is to get my prescriptions in… I got nothing really to go up there for and there's always a surgery full of people in a far worse state than you, so no I don't bother them at all… that's life for me" (male, age 80)

Furthermore, several respondents stated that, before they had considered themselves a TJR candidate, they felt they had to be in constant pain or almost incapacitated. As such, surgery was viewed as the last resort:

> "…but it depends on how crippled you get, you know, I think you get to your last resort where you will try anything to be able to walk properly" (male, age 70)

9.3.2
Age and Candidacy for Surgery

In C.S.'s study, several respondents assumed that they would not be considered as appropriate candidates for surgery because they believed they would be considered "too old" for surgery. As a result, they did not feel it was worthwhile consulting their GP or having a referral to a hospital consultant:

> "Well I think, I do think to myself I shall be 90 next year. Perhaps all that money they might spend on me could be done perhaps for a younger person. That's the way I'm looking at

it. Also, I'm wondering if they put me on a list, it would be so long a wait, it probably wouldn't be worth it. I don't know if they do you when you get so old" (female, age 89)

This reluctance to seek treatment also stemmed from perceptions of the risks and personal costs of surgery. In G.W.'s study, the respondents who were on the waiting list for surgery often used positive stories about people with favourable outcomes to support their own decisions to have surgery. However, in C.S.'s study, the majority of respondents knew other people who had had joint replacements, but because many reported poor outcomes, particularly from knee surgery, they were fearful, or at least uncertain, about whether or not they should submit to having surgery themselves:

"…to be quite honest, so many of my friends that I know have had, they haven't been satisfactory. I mean one after 3 years her knee completely went again, and another one had never been free of pain since after going through with the surgery. So, I thought, well if I can manage without it, you know, I would" (female, age 83)

9.3.3
Lay Beliefs of TJR

A theme to emerge from the data in G.W.'s study was the informants' perception of the effectiveness of TKR. Total hip replacement was seen as a more effective operation than TKR, suggesting that many people in the UK still regard knee replacements as being more experimental. However, despite the fact that TKRs were seen as inferior to THRs, attitudes towards TKR seemed to be slowly changing: the majority of the informants believed that there had been improvements in TKR in the past decades. This may reflect an improvement in TKR operations or may reveal the informants' optimistic view of a good outcome for themselves:

"…and of course I do believe the knee operation… years ago I wouldn't have it, no way, because they said the hip was good but the knees weren't too good… they have improved over the years I believe but years ago they weren't so sure of the knees so I used to say I'd never have my knees done… of course when you get to such pain… I feel a lot different now" (female, age 80)

9.3.4
Weight, Co-morbidity and Personal Factors

A number of personal factors leading to reluctance to have surgery were identified in C.S.'s study, such as weight, co-morbidity (such as more pressing heart problems) or responsibilities such as caring for a spouse:

"…if they're going to do something like that, my wife, where is she going to be like, do you know what I mean?… I wouldn't put her away or anything like, no" (male, age 74)

These views were expressed by older respondents; the four youngest people were much more determined to get treatment. They were all of working age and three were in paid employment. Three had found it necessary to pay for a private referral to a specialist.

9.3.5
Influence of Physicians on Assessments of Need and Timing

Respondents stated clearly in C.S.'s study that they did not want to "bother" community physicians with symptoms for which they considered there was no appropriate/acceptable treatment. For some, the community physicians seemed to reinforce the perception that nothing could be done:

> "I've told him the doctor (about joint problems) and he said "well there's nothing really we can do about it", and well I just say it's something I've just got to put up with and get on with" (female, age 91)

Even for those individuals on the waiting list for TKR, a minority of community physicians also expressed concerns about the effectiveness of the TKR procedure and the risk of revision operations. Furthermore, in both studies, several reported that community physicians had informed them that they were not suitable candidates for surgery:

> "I was in agonies and um, I said to him [doctor] 'what about me knees being done?', and he said 'look Mrs X, if it was your hips I would send you in, but they don't do the knees much good, they're not perfect with it'. He said "you're wasting your money to have a specialist"" (female, age 82)

9.3.6
Differing Priorities Between Patients and Physicians

The respondents in G.W.'s study discussed their views about the consultants' decision to list for surgery and raised issues concerning the priority and indications for surgery in general. They thought that decisions for TKR were being made according to a number of factors, such as weight and age. Several respondents were told that their excess weight was a problem; many of them felt that this was unfair and that the doctors did not appreciate that arthritis led to reduced mobility and therefore to weight gain:

> "All I was told was to lose a bit of weight and come back again which, like I said, just annoys me a little bit, well a lot really, because I have had all the problems before I put the weight on... since then I've given up the sport and I've been doing less and less physical exercise I have put the weight on... They tend to look at you as thought it is your own fault... the problems I have got have not been caused by being overweight... I'm overweight because of the problems that I've got" (male, age 48)

Others thought that age was used as a criterion. Respondents felt that they needed TJR, but believed that they had been stalled from having the surgery because the surgeon considered them to be "too young"

9

"I said, 'well can I have something done about it, can I have an operation?' And they said, 'No, you are too young'... I think there should be some way, irrespective of age. I would rather go in and have a check up every 10 years than endure the pain... so if this could be done earlier, you are not like this... I should be out now enjoying myself because I have worked hard all my life" (female, age 75)

A small, but perhaps important group felt that the system was unfair in other ways. For example, some were sure that knowing or bothering the surgeon (and excessive complaining) could result in earlier treatment and others were concerned that private care meant that some received unfair earlier treatment, with two believing that "foreigners" were also seen too early.

9.4
Discussion

This chapter reports on two independent studies carried out to explore patients' views of TJR in the UK; they explore the views of individuals who have been both successful and unsuccessful in being referred to the TJR waiting list. The first study (C.S.) explored barriers to health care utilisation in respondents with moderate/severe hip/knee disease in the community and clearly identified unmet need. The second study (G.W.) examined the views of individuals on the waiting list for TJR and revealed their perceived views on surgical priority. Both studies demonstrate that views of consumers about appropriateness of surgery are complex. The key finding is that older people are often reluctant to put themselves forward for treatment for a variety of reasons. Moreover, when they do try to access formal care and treatment, they experience several barriers.

The "normalisation" of arthritis appears to a major factor in health care utilisation. The interview data in both studies demonstrated that older respondents play down the significance of their symptoms because of their age and are therefore pessimistic and reluctant to seek formal health care. These findings are consistent with the findings of previous research [13, 14]. Furthermore, the risks and personal costs of surgery were represented in stories told by respondents about people they knew (or had heard about) who had already had surgery. Those respondents who had received surgery, or were on the waiting list for surgery, often used positive stories about people with favourable outcomes to support their own decisions to have surgery. For respondents who were undecided about surgery, stories of good and bad outcomes seemed to add to and reflect their uncertainty.

Knee replacement surgery was presented as the more "risky" procedure and this may have hindered some of the informants' decision to seek help. Many respondents recounted discussions with community physicians about the risks and benefits of surgery, which seemed to have an important influence on decision-making. Their experiences were mostly negative, with doctors appearing to confirm the lack of effective treatment.

Waiting lists and rationing were also perceived to be a barrier to getting treatment in secondary care, and sometimes TJR appeared to be denied because they were considered "too young", or overweight. However, there is no evidence to suggest that operating on obese or older patients leads to more failures or complications [15, 16]. Recent research has suggested that patients with the most severe disease at the time of TKR improved to a similar degree to those operated on earlier, meaning that they never "caught up" with those who were less disabled at the time of TKR [17]. These data also show that the oldest people having an operation usually benefit a great deal, but not as much as younger people.

Several approaches need to be addressed with regard to unmet need and the perceived prioritisation of TJR. There is a need for information to counter prevalent lay beliefs that arthritis is an untreatable and inevitable part of ageing. Practitioners may have to initiate these discussions, since many older people are often reliant on their practitioners to provide information about their health care. Consequently, for this to be successful, information about TKR as an effective procedure also needs to be disseminated among GPs and the public. There also needs to be a debate about appropriate indications for TJR, and particularly the importance of factors such as age and obesity.

References

1. Williams MH, Frankel S, Nanchahal K, Coast J, Donovan J. Total Hip Replacement. In: Stevens A, Raftery J, eds. Health Care Needs Assessment, Oxford: Radcliffe Medical Press, 1994, pp. 448–523
2. Mancuso CA, Ranawat CS, Esdaile JM, Johanson NA, Charlson ME. Indications for total hip and knee arthroplasties. The Journal of Arthroplasty 1996. 11: 34–46
3. Wright JG, Coyte P, Hawker G, et al. Variation in orthopaedic surgeons' perceptions of the indications for and outcomes of knee replacement. Canadian Medical Association Journal 1995. 152: 687–697
4. Birrell F, Johnell O, Silman A. Projecting the need for hip replacement over the next three decades: influence of changing demography and threshold for surgery. Annals of the Rheumatic Diseases 1999. 58: 569–572
5. Tennant A, Fear J, Pickering A, Hillman M, Cutts A, Chamberlain MA. Prevalence of knee problems in the population aged 55 years and over: identifying the need for knee arthroplasty. British Medical Journal 1995. 310: 1291–1293
6. Dieppe P, Basler HD, Chard J, et al. Knee replacement surgery for osteoarthritis: effectiveness, practice variations, indications and possible determinants of utilization. British Journal of Rheumatology 1999. 38: 73–83
7. Katz BP, Freund DA, Heck D, et al. Demographic variation in the rate of knee replacement: a multi-year analysis. Health Services Research 1996. 31: 125–140
8. Chaturvedi N, Ben-Shlomo Y. From the surgery to the surgeon: does deprivation influence consultation and operation rates? British Journal of General Practice 1995. 45: 127–131
9. Hawker GA, Wright JG, Coyte PC, et al. Differences between men and women in the rate of use of hip and knee arthroplasty. New England Journal of Medicine 2000. 342: 1016–1022
10. Pope C, Mays N. Reaching the parts other methods cannot reach: an introduction to qualitative methods in health and health services research. British Medical Journal 1995. 311: 42–45
11. Malterud K. Qualitative research: standards, challenges, and guidelines. The Lancet 2001. 358: 483–488
12. Glaser BG, Strauss AL. The discovery of grounded theory. Chicago: Aldine, 1967
13. Blaxter M. The causes of disease. Women talking. Social Science and Medicine 1983. 17: 59–69
14. Hudak PL, Clark JP, Hawker GA, et al. "You're perfect for the procedure! Why don't you want it" Elderly arthritis patients' unwillingness to consider total joint arthroplasty surgery: a qualitative study. Medical Decision Making 2002. 22: 272–278
15. Griffin FM, Scuderi GR, Insall JN, Colizza W. Total knee arthroplasty in patients who were obese with 10 years follow up. Clinical Orthopaedics and Related Research 1998. 356: 28–33
16. Donell S, Neyret P, Dejour H, Adeleine P. The effect of age on the quality of life after knee replacement. Knee 1998. 5: 125–128
17. Kennedy LG, Newman JH, Ackroyd CE, Dieppe P. Are our patients waiting too long for their knee replacements? Rheumatology 2001. Suppl 1: 73(Abstract)

Population Requirement for Primary Hip-Replacement Surgery in England: A Comparison with Knee-Replacement

10

P. Jüni and P. Dieppe

10.1
Introduction

The debate about health care rationing, in terms of both its justification and mechanism, is conducted largely in the absence of data. The relevant literature mainly consists of assertion, exploration of ethical principles and political analysis. In particular, an epidemiological basis for the assumption that demand for effective treatments will invariably exceed supply is lacking. Waiting list figures suggest that health services are not satisfying demand in particular areas, but this does not mean that demand is generally insatiable.

Total hip and knee replacements are effective interventions for patients with severe joint disease, resulting in large improvements in patient-related outcome measures for the majority of those undergoing these procedures. Although the number of operations performed in England has been rising each year over the last two decades [1], it has been suggested that there is still a large unmet need. However, the current evidence base is limited. Some prevalence data on severe joint disease in the community are available [2], but incidence data to estimate the annual population requirement for hip and knee replacement are lacking. Consensus criteria for case selection for total joint replacement (TJR) have been published [3, 4], but data on the impact of these criteria on annual rates are unavailable, and the implications of different thresholds for surgery, patient preference and other modifiers of the decision to recommend surgery are unclear.

We used prevalence data from the Somerset and Avon Survey of Health (SASH) [5–7] to estimate the annual population requirement for primary hip and knee replacement in England, also comparing health care utilisation by people with hip and knee disease.

P. Juni (✉)
Institute of Social and Preventive Medicine, Universität Bern,
Finkenhubelweg 11, 3012, Bern, Switzerland
e-mail: juni@ispm.unibe.ch

K.E. Dreinhöfer et al. (eds.), *EUROHIP: Health Technology Assessment of Hip Arthroplasty in Europe*, DOI: 10.1007/978-3-540-74137-4_10, © 2009 EFORT

10.2
Patients and Methods

10.2.1
Sampling of Patients

SASH is a population-based cross-sectional study described elsewhere [5, 7]. We used a multistage sampling strategy [8]. Forty general practices were selected from Avon and Somerset; from each practice, 702 people aged 35 years and over were randomly selected using age/sex stratification, resulting in a sample of 28,080 people with the numbers of men and women in each 10-year age band reflecting the population distribution of Avon and Somerset [5]. After exclusion of 2,034 people who had moved out of the study area, suffered from a severe mental illness or a terminal illness, or were deceased, 26,046 people were included in the study. Approval was obtained from the relevant ethics committees [7].

10.2.2
Screening Process

All 26,046 people were sent a screening questionnaire comprising questions on general health, utilisation of health services and symptoms of hip and knee disease. Non-respondents were sent two reminders and contacted by telephone, if necessary [5]. We screened people for hip and knee pain using a modified version of the questions used in the first National Health and Nutrition Examination Survey [9]: "During the past twelve months, have you had pain in or around either of your hips (knees) on most days for one month or longer?" Participants who reported hip or knee pain were invited for further examination either at a clinic or by home visit. Examinations were organised in two phases by location of participating practices.

10.2.3
Orthopaedic Assessment

Interviewer-administered questionnaires were completed on hip and knee pain and stiffness, activities of daily living, use of health services and referral to specialist care. Participants were asked whether they had received drug therapy for their joint pain in the previous year, whether they suffered from symptoms that might make them unfit for surgery (chest tightness, wheeze, breathlessness, chest pain or palpitations), and whether they would accept surgery if it were offered, with a follow-up question to elicit the reasons for their view. A clinical examination of hip, knee and lower back was carried out by a physician and a team of nurses with orthopaedic experience who had undergone a standard training programme.

10.2.4
Criteria for Case Selection

The New Zealand priority criteria for major joint replacement surgery [4] (New Zealand Score) were used for case selection for primary TJR. In a pilot study, agreement of the developed criteria with overall clinical judgement was found to be excellent [10]. The final composite score included sub-scores on pain (40 points), disability (20 points), clinical findings (20 points), and multiple joint disease and ability to live independently (20 points), and ranged from 0 to 100 with higher scores reflecting more severe disease. No agreed cut-off point for case selection were proposed. To reflect severe and moderate disease, we chose a priori threshold scores of 55 (primary cut-off) and 43 (secondary cut-off), respectively. Examples for degrees of pain and disability associated with these cut-off points have been published previously [7].

10.2.5
Statistical Methods

Incidence and prevalence calculations were carried out in an identical way for hip and knee disease [6, 7]. We calculated age- and sex-specific prevalence of already replaced joints for those responding to the screening questionnaire. Then we estimated the prevalence of joint disease warranting TJR (cut-off points 43 and 55 on the New Zealand Score) using extrapolations from the examined group of participants to the overall group reporting symptoms with age/sex-specific sampling fractions and the assumption that attendees and non-attendees were similar. New Zealand Scores were not assigned to joints which had already been replaced.

Incidence was calculated by the method of Leske et al. [11], using the increase in prevalence between consecutive age bands to calculate age-specific incidence. Its assumptions have been discussed before [7]. We considered prevalence data for replaced and severely diseased joints (New Zealand Scores ≥43 or 55 points) separately and smoothed both by fitting quadratic models across age-groups in logistic regression analysis. Then, we included age/sex-specific death rates. The annual number of TJRs needed in the population of England was calculated by multiplying point estimates and 95% confidence intervals of age/sex-specific incidences by population figures for England. This number was modified by excluding those assumed to be unfit for surgery (self-reported chest tightness, wheeze, breathlessness, chest pain or palpitations many times a day or all the time), those who had not had a trial of medical therapy in the past year, and those who indicated they might not accept surgery if offered it.

For exploratory analyses, we defined index joints as the symptomatic hip or knee with the highest New Zealand score (1,302 index hips and 2,056 index knees). We used logistic regression models to compare the use of health services and referral to specialist care for knee versus hip disease, using robust standard errors, which allowed for correlation within participants who suffered from both knee and hip disease, and adjusting for disease severity. In a further analysis, we also adjusted for age, gender, and willingness and fitness for surgery; because of missing data, this analysis was based on 2,928 index joints only. Finally, we extracted the annual number of primary total hip and knee replacements performed in English NHS hospitals from first episodes of 1997 Hospital Episode Statistics [1]. The number of procedures performed independently was estimated using data from a 1997 national survey of private hospitals in England [12].

10.3
Results

A total of 22,978 individuals responded to the screening questionnaire, 22,217 completed the question on hip pain and 22,379 the question on knee pain. A total of 6,416 participants reported hip or knee pain, or both (28.7%). Of those, 4,304 were invited for further examination either at a clinic or by home visit (67.1%) and 2,703 attended (62.8%). Prevalence of joint pain increased with age and was higher in women than in men [5, 6]. Attendees were more likely than non-attendees to have sought care for joint disease [5, 6].

The prevalence of primary TJRs was 22.0 joints per 1,000 people aged 35 years and over for hips (95% CI 20.1–24.0), and 8.4 joints per 1,000 people for knees (95% CI 7.2–9.5). Using the primary cut-off of 55 points on the New Zealand Score, we found an estimated population prevalence of hip disease requiring TJR of 18.2 joints per 1,000 people aged 35 years and over (95% CI 16.0–21.2), increasing to 36.5 with a cut-off of 43 points (95% CI 34.0–40.8). Respective figures for knee disease were 27.4 joints per 1,000 people aged 35 years and over (95% CI 24.7–30.1), increasing to 64.3 with a cut-off of 43 points (95% CI 60.8–67.7).

Prevalence figures translated into an estimated incidence of 54,000 hips (95% CI 35,900–72,100) for a cut-off of 55 points, and 64,800 hips for a cut-off of 43 points (95% CI 44,600–85,000), respectively, requiring total hip replacement annually in England. The annual number of primary total hip replacements actually performed in England in 1997 were 31,300 in the NHS [1] and an additional estimated 10,100 in independent hospitals [12]. Figure 10.1 shows respective numbers for knees for a cut-off of 55 points and the effect on estimates for hip and knee replacements when suitability for surgery and patients' preferences were accounted for, comparing hips with knees [6]. The number of hips requiring TJR in England decreased only moderately to 46,200 after exclusion of those people who were unfit for surgery, had not had a trial of medical therapy, or indicated they did not want a surgical intervention (95% CI 27,500–64,900). In contrast, the number of knees requiring TJRs decreased to about half of the initial estimate after using the same criteria for exclusion of people unsuitable or unfit for surgery (29,100, 95% CI 16,300–41,900). Willingness to consider surgery had a greater impact on incidence estimates for knees than of hips, indicating that patients may be more reluctant to undergo knee replacement than hip replacement. After adjustment for severity of disease, those with hip disease were less likely than those with knee disease to have sought care from their GP [odds ratio (OR) 0.78, 95% CI 0.66–0.93), but more likely to have been referred to specialist care (OR 1.23, 95% CI 1.04–1.45), to have consulted an orthopaedic surgeon (OR 1.42, 95% CI 1.09–1.86), or to be on a waiting list for joint replacement (OR 2.39, 95% CI 1.22–4.68).

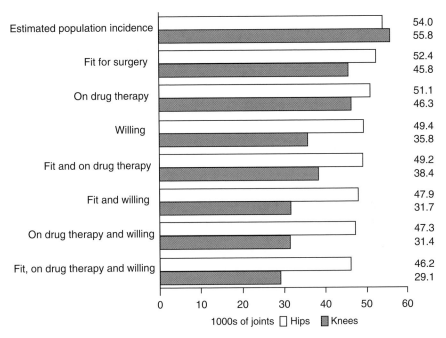

Fig. 10.1 Estimated annual number of incident hip and knee disease requiring primary total joint replacement surgery for those aged 35–85 years in England. Expressed as 1,000s of joints required in England

Differences remained after additional adjustment for age, gender, willingness and fitness for surgery [6].

10.4
Discussion

The majority of people with hip and knee pain do not suffer from severe disease. A variety of outcome instruments are available to help grade the severity of symptoms, such as Lequesne's index [13] or WOMAC [14], but these instruments were not developed for case selection for TJR. In contrast, the priority criteria from Ontario, Canada [3], and New Zealand [4] were produced for this very reason. The New Zealand priority criteria provide a numerical score which can be used to define indications for surgery from population-based data [5]. Using these criteria, we calculated the prevalence of hip and knee disease severe enough to warrant TJR. However, interventions such as TJR are provided on an incident basis, so we converted prevalence figures to incidence data. Using the primary cut-off point this translated to a calculated annual need for 54,000 total hip replacements and 55,800 total knee replacements. When estimates were adjusted for potential modifiers of the decision to recommend surgery (fitness, willingness and previous drug therapy), the incidence estimates decreased to approximately 75% for hip replacements and 50% for

10

knee replacements. Resulting estimates of 46,200 hips and 29,100 knees requiring TJR annually corresponded approximately to the observed 41,400 hips and 29,300 knees actually replaced in England in 1997.

Rates vary greatly in different countries [15]. Surprisingly, the actually observed provision of total hip replacements exceeds the rates found in the USA [16], where adequate provision is assumed: 52 per 100,000 of the overall population, corresponding to about 32,000 operations that would be performed annually in England. In contrast, the observed provision of knee replacements amounts to only 50% of that observed in the USA, 92 per 100,000 of the overall population, corresponding to about 58,000 operations performed annually in England.

We also found interesting differences between hip and knee disease in the pattern of health services utilisation along the whole pathway to joint replacement, with a lower provision of care for knee disease. Referral patterns by primary care physicians may be of particular importance. Differences remained, however, when we adjusted for referral to specialist care, indicating that differential provision of care may also be an issue at the level of specialists. Part of this difference may be due to the fact that hip disease often deteriorates rapidly, with a relatively sudden increase in the level of pain [17], while knee disease usually deteriorates slowly, giving patients and physicians more time to adjust to and accept increasing severity [15].

The limitations of our approach to estimate population requirements for joint replacement were discussed previously [6, 7]. Despite these limitations, our data suggest that there is at most only a moderate underprovision of total hip replacements, but a considerable underprovision of total knee replacements in England. Our study indicates that this may not simply be due to a failure of the National Health System to satisfy demand, but also because of reluctance by patients and doctors to consider surgery in some instances. While the satisfaction of demand for total hip replacement, given agreed criteria, appears to be a realistic objective in England, a review of policies for the management of knee disease is needed.

Acknowledgements We thank all study participants and the partners and staff of participating general practices for their support and interest in the study. We are indebted to the whole of the SASH research team: Kirsty Alchin, Ros Berkeley-Hill, Jane Brooks, Hilary Brownett, Phil Chan, Clare Cross, Catherine Dawe, Cathy Doel, Jenny Eachus, Helen Forward, Matthew Grainge, Rosemary Greenwood, Fiona Hollyman, Sue Jones, Helen Moore, Kate Morris, Nicky Pearson, Brian Quilty, Chris Smith, Lynne Smith, Gwyn Williams, Mark Williams, Sue Williams, and Andrea Wilson; and Allan Douglas and Doreen Cook at Dillon Computing. Finally, we are grateful to our co-investigators, Jenny Donovan, Tim Peters and Stephen Frankel, and to Brian Williams for providing unpublished data. The SASH was originally funded by the Department of Health and the South and West NHS Research and Development Directorate. This work was funded by the Swiss National Science Foundation (grants no. 3233-066377 and 3200-066378). The Department of Social Medicine is the lead centre for the MRC Health Services Research Collaboration.

References

1. Hospital episode statistics 1997. London: Department of Health, 1998
2. Tennant A, Fear J, Pickering A, Hillman M, Cutts A, Chamberlain MA. Prevalence of knee problems in the population aged 55 years and over: identifying the need for knee arthroplasty. BMJ 1995; 310:1291–1293
3. Taylor CD, Williams JI. Primary hip and knee replacement surgery: Ontario criteria for case selection and surgical priority. Qual Health Care 1996; 5:20–30
4. Hadorn DC, Holmes AC. The New Zealand priority criteria project. Part 1: overview. BMJ 1997; 314:131–134
5. Eachus J, Williams M, Chan P, Smith GD, Grainge M, Donovan J, Frankel S. Deprivation and cause specific morbidity: evidence from the Somerset and Avon survey of health. BMJ 1996; 312:287–292
6. Jüni P, Dieppe P, Donovan J, Peters T, Eachus J, Pearson N, Greenwood R, Frankel S. Population requirement for primary knee replacement surgery: a cross-sectional study. Rheumatology 2003; 42:516–521
7. Frankel S, Eachus J, Pearson N, Greenwood R, Chan P, Peters TJ, Donovan J, Smith GD, Dieppe P. Population requirement for primary hip-replacement surgery: a cross-sectional study. Lancet 1999; 353:1304–1309
8. Peters TJ, Eachus JI. Achieving equal probability of selection under various random sampling strategies. Paediatr Perinat Epidemiol 1995; 9:219–224
9. Anderson JJ, Felson DT. Factors associated with osteoarthritis of the knee in the first national Health and Nutrition Examination Survey (HANES I). Evidence for an association with overweight, race, and physical demands of work. Am J Epidemiol 1988; 128:179–189
10. Hadorn DC, Holmes A. The New Zealand Priority Criteria Project. Criteria Pilot Tests. Available at:http://www.bmj.com/cgi/content/full/314/7074/131/DC1. Accessed December 12, 2001
11. Leske MC, Ederer F, Podgor M. Estimating incidence from age-specific prevalence in glaucoma. Am J Epidemiol 1981; 113:606–613
12. Williams B, Whatmough P, McGill J, Rushton L. Private funding of elective hospital treatment in England and Wales, 1997–1998: national survey. BMJ 2000; 320:904–905
13. Lequesne MG, Mery C, Samson M, Gerard P. Indexes of severity for osteoarthritis of the hip and knee. Scand J Rheumatol Suppl 1987; 65:85–89
14. Bellamy N, Buchanan WW, Goldsmith CH, Campbell J, Stitt LW. Validation study of WOMAC: a health status instrument for measuring clinically important patient relevant outcomes following total hip or knee arthroplasty in osteoarthritis. J Orthop Rheumatol 1988; 1:95–108
15. Dieppe P, Basler HD, Chard J, Croft P, Dixon J, Hurley M, Lohmander S, Raspe H. Knee replacement surgery for osteoarthritis: effectiveness, practice variations, indications and possible determinants of utilization. Rheumatology (Oxford) 1999; 38:73–83
16. National hospital discharge survey 1997. Hyattsville, Maryland: National Center for Health Statistics, 1998
17. Dougados M, Gueguen A, Nguyen M, Berdah L, Lequesne M, Mazieres B, Vignon E. Radiological progression of hip osteoarthritis: definition, risk factors and correlations with clinical status. Ann Rheum Dis 1996; 55:356–362

Part III

Outcome Measurement

What Are the Outcomes After Hip Joint Replacement for OA?

11

L.S. Lohmander

Total hip replacement (THR) is an effective intervention with a good cost/benefit ratio. Worldwide, each year it brings relief in the form of improved function and decreased pain to at least half a million patients with severe osteoarthritis (OA). Since the introduction by Charnley more than 30 years ago, the basic concept remains much the same, but with a multitude of changes in details of surgical procedure and implant design. Some changes have been introduced after careful testing and controlled trials, many of them without. In spite of this, the experience of most large follow-up series, including the Scandinavian national implant registries, show a gradual improvement in the success rate of THR with increased surgeon experience and improved procedures [7].

The outcome of THR for OA in these large-scale follow-up series is usually measured in terms of implant survival, or failure rate usually defined as reoperation, and is calculated by Kaplan–Meier life table statistics. As indicated by the terminology, this outcome focusses on the fate of the implant, but to a large extent ignores the experience of the patient, which can be inferred only indirectly and distantly through these statistics. Nevertheless, much valuable information has been gained through national implant registries such as that for THR run continuously since 1979 in Sweden, now having registered more than 200,000 primary THR procedures [7]. Measured by this technique, the 10-year implant failure rate of the average modern cemented hip implant due to aseptic loosening (the major reason for reoperation) is now about 5% in Sweden. Failure rates for uncemented implants, for young patients and for patients operated in the beginning of the THR era, are two to three times higher. The peri-operative mortality is comparable with other surgical procedures, and long-term mortality actually lower than for the average age-matched population, perhaps due to a "healthy-patient" selection for THR [6]. Through the registries in Sweden and the other Nordic countries, the more suboptimal THR designs and procedures have been identified early after introduction and their use discouraged through reports back to the users [2, 3].

L.S. Lohmander (✉)
Department of Orthopedics, Lund University, Lund University Hospital,
22185 Lund, Sweden
e-mail: stefan.lohmander@med.lu.se

K.E. Dreinhöfer et al. (eds.), *EUROHIP: Health Technology Assessment*
of Hip Arthroplasty in Europe, DOI: 10.1007/978-3-540-74137-4_11, © 2009 EFORT

11 As mentioned, many modifications in THR designs and procedures have been introduced over the years, often with limited testing and lack of controlled trials, and sometimes to the detriment of the THR patient [2]. Although the nation-wide registries can serve to identify inferior designs and procedures without too much delay once they have reached the market, they cannot prevent the initial marketing and use of such inferior designs. With the considerable success of current THR procedures, and generally low implant failure rates, very large and very long-term controlled trials are required to show superiority, or even non-inferiority, of a new implant over the comparator implant. Such trials are thus really not a viable route to further improvements in THR outcome, being too costly and too time consuming. They would, in addition, expose large numbers of patients to a new implant of unknown benefit.

Radiological methods, and in particular radiostereometry (radiostereometric analysis, RSA), have been suggested as a way to precisely monitor implant migration, thus being able to compare exactly the movement over time of two different implants. With use of this technology, it becomes feasible to compare different implants, exposing a limited number of patients over a limited time to the new procedure [4]. However, this requires that short-term implant migration or wear is a valid surrogate outcome for long-term implant failure rate. There is as yet only limited published evidence for this [10], and even less support for it being a valid surrogate endpoint for the clinical endpoint of patient-relevant outcome.

The purpose of THR for OA is to decrease pain and to maintain or improve function and quality of life for the patient. The outcome as experienced and scored by the patient should thus be the gold standard (clinical endpoint) against which measures such as implant migration or survival are validated (Table 11.1). Until such validation has been proven, these outcomes remain by definition "measures", with an uncertain connection to the clinical endpoint. It is only after validation that the measure can be considered a surrogate endpoint to serve in place of a clinical endpoint. The basic question needing an answer is: how well does the measure or surrogate endpoint reflect patient preference and quality of life (Fig. 11.1)? We also need to recognize that beneficial effects of treatment may occur via pathways that do not include the surrogate measure being monitored. Further, surrogates do not always account for adverse effects which may cancel out all or part of an apparent treatment benefit.

While investigations that focus on outcomes such as implant survival have successfully identified a number of important variables related to, e.g. implant, cement, procedure and surgeon, patient-related factors other than age or sex that influence outcome after THR have received comparatively little attention. Not surprisingly, published data show that

Table 11.1 The relationship between a surrogate endpoint and a clinical endpoint

Clinical endpoint	A characteristic or variable that measures how a patient feels, functions or survives
Measure, marker	Measured and evaluated as an indicator of a biological or pathological process, or response to a therapeutic intervention
Surrogate endpoint	A measure or marker intended to substitute for a clinical endpoint

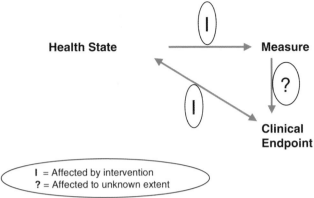

Intervention affects endpoint and measure independently
An unknown proportion of intervention effect is captured by measure

Fig. 11.1 A surrogate measure rarely captures the full effect of the intervention, be it a positive or a negative one

"failure rates" of implants are much higher when measured as, e.g. pain than as implant revision rate, reinforcing the need for routine use of patient-relevant outcome measures to complement implant-related outcomes [1]. However, few long-term studies of patient-relevant outcome after THR for OA have been published.

It is thus of interest to note that a long-term, community-based, prospective and consecutive follow-up after THR for OA showed that hip OA patients over 50 years of age at 3.6 years after unilateral THR reported similar pain, but experienced a lower level of physical function, than a matched reference group without hip complaints [9]. The study included a matched reference group and well-validated patient-relevant outcome instruments. The difference in function was explained at least in part by the presence of musculoskeletal co-morbidities such as low back pain and pain in the non-operated hip. The majority of the patients experienced a significant improvement in pain and function after THR. However, at 3.6 years after surgery, almost one-third of the patients reported only a low degree of improvement or having deteriorated in pain and/or function following the THR. Part of this lack of response may be explained by old age and a high degree of pain at the time of surgery. A report of low back pain had a significant impact on postoperative function after THR. However, the influence on outcome by the radiological stage of the hip OA at the time of surgery is very limited [8]. It was recently shown that hospital and surgeon volume significantly influenced patient satisfaction after THR, even after adjusting for sociodemographic and clinical variables: satisfaction was greater among patients who underwent primary THR in large-volume centres [5]. However, there was no influence on patient-reported functional status.

It is clear that even after identifying these predictors, a major proportion of the variability in outcome after THR for OA remains unexplained. Further patient-relevant outcome data

11

collected by the use of self-administered questionnaires, and a better understanding of the role of expectations and satisfaction, is essential to improve our understanding of who does or does not benefit from these surgical procedures. Such data would have their greatest utility if they were collected in a manner that allowed linking to large implant registries. Much effort is focussed on the "technical" aspects of the THR intervention to further improve its success rate. Perhaps we may stand to gain as much or more in THR outcome improvement by a better understanding of the "other" factors. Finally, our views on what are the most relevant outcome measures will likely influence how we assess needs for THR.

References

1. Britton AR, Murray DW, Bulstrode CJ, McPherson K, Denham RA. Pain levels after total hip replacement: their use as endpoints for survival analysis. J Bone Joint Surg Br 1997;79:93–98
2. Espehaug B, Fumes O, Havelin LI, Engesaeter LB, Vollset SE. The type of cement and failure of total hip replacements. J Bone Joint Surg Br 2002;84:832–838
3. Herberts P, Malchau H. Long-term registration has improved the quality of hip replacement: a review of the Swedish THR Register comparing 160,000 cases. Acta Orthop Scand 2000;71:111–121
4. Kärrholm J, Anderberg C, Snorrason F, Thanner J, Langeland N, Malchau H, Herberts P. Evaluation of a femoral stem with reduced stiffness. A randomized study with use of radiosteo-reometry and bone densitometry. J Bone Joint Surg Am 2002;84-A:1651–1658
5. Katz JN, Phillips CB, Baron JA, Fossel AH, Mahomed NN, Barrett J, Lingard EA, Harris WH, Poss R, Lew RA, Guadagnoli E, Wright EA, Losina E. Association of hospital and surgeon volume of total hip replacement with functional status and satisfaction three years following surgery. Arthritis Rheum 2003;48:560–568
6. Lie SA, Engesaeter LB, Havelin LI, Furnes O, Vollset SE. Early postoperative mortality after 67,548 total hip replacements: causes of death and thromboprophylaxis in 68 hospitals in Norway from 1987 to 1999. Acta Orthop Scand 2002;73:392–399
7. Malchau H, Herberts P, Eisler T, Garellick G, Söderman P. The Swedish total hip replacement register. J Bone Joint Surg Am 2002;84-A Suppl 2:2–20
8. Nilsdotter AK, Aurell Y, Siösteen AK, Lohmander LS, Roos HP. Radiographic stage of osteoarthritis or sex does not predict one year outcome after total hip arthroplasty. Ann Rheum Dis 2001;60:228–232
9. Nilsdotter A-K, Petersson IF, Roos EM, Lohmander LS. Predictors of patient-relevant outcome after total hip replacement for osteoarthritis – a prospective study. Ann Rheum Dis 2003;62:923–930
10. Ryd L, Albrektsson BE, Carlsson L, Dansgard F, Herberts P, Lindstrand A, Regner L, Toksvig-Larsen S. Roentgen stereophotogrammetric analysis as a predictor of mechanical loosening of knee prostheses. J Bone Joint Surg Br 1995;77:377–383

Outcomes of Hip Replacement Vary

12

A. Nilsdotter

12.1
The Definition of a Result

It is not obvious how we should define a satisfactory result after total hip replacement. The result can be defined as the absolute change, the degree of improvement or the absolute outcome score level the patient reaches. Two of these definitions are dependent on the baseline status. The first definition has the disadvantage of presenting a non-satisfactory result in patients who are not as disabled at baseline as patients who are more disabled. On the other hand, it is important to recognize that patients with a relatively good status at baseline do not have the possibility to improve as much as the others.

12.2
Individual Change

It has previously been shown [1] that about 10% of the patients who receive a total hip replacement do not improve in pain and function at a 1-year follow-up (Fig. 12.1). These results were confirmed in a study published in 2002 [2]. In an intermediate follow-up of patients 3.6 years after total hip replacement, as many as 31% of the patients had not improved more than 10 score units (minimal perceptible clinical improvement) in WOMAC pain and/or function on a 0–100 scale [3] It is not evident that these patients are the same as the patients who are classified as failures when you use prosthesis survival as endpoint [4]. Not very much attention has been paid to the group of patients that do not improve, apart from the ones with prosthetic and technical failures.

A. Nilsdotter (✉)
Department of Research and Education, Halmstad Central Hospital, 301 85 Halmstad, Sweden
e-mail: Anna.Nilsdotter@lthalland.se

K.E. Dreinhöfer et al. (eds.), *EUROHIP: Health Technology Assessment*
of Hip Arthroplasty in Europe, DOI: 10.1007/978-3-540-74137-4_12, © 2009 EFORT

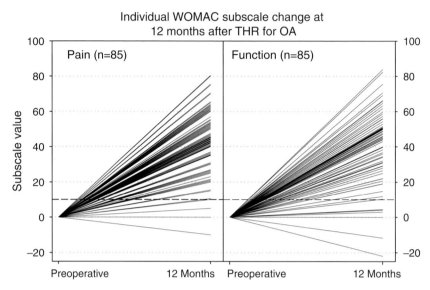

Fig. 12.1 Individual change in WOMAC pain and function following THR calculated as the difference between preoperative and postoperative score at 12 months. Each *line* represents one patient

12.3
Why Does Outcome Vary?

12.3.1
Age

The importance of age has been investigated thoroughly. It has been shown that age is important for the postoperative outcome in physical function where the younger patients reach a better absolute average score than the older. The degree of improvement (expressed in score points) in physical function is also greater for the younger than the older patients. In a recent study [2], there was no difference in the experience of postoperative pain at 1 year between younger and older patients. That finding is in agreement with a previous study [5].

When defining an unsatisfying result as the patients who scored worst (lowest quartile) in WOMAC function at an intermediate follow-up, age was found to be a predictor for poor outcome. However, age does not seem to be of significance for the degree of relieving pain. Independent of age pain relief is experienced very soon after surgery, while the adaptation to the new health status as expressed by the SF-36 dimension RP(role function) takes at least 12 months. This is in accordance with previous studies where gains in pain improvement were found to be faster than gains in physical function [6].

12.3.2
Gender

Women have been shown to experience a higher degree of preoperative pain than men in connection with THR [7], while another study found no gender differences in either prosthesis survival or quality of life [6]. When analysing 198 patients at an intermediate follow-up after total hip replacement, there was no difference between the sexes in WOMAC outcome, nor was there any difference in their preoperative values [3].

Because of the divergent findings it is difficult to draw any conclusions. If there is a real preoperative difference, it may be due to female–male differences in pain responses. Postoperatively, however, there does not seem to be any difference between the sexes.

12.3.3
Co-morbidities

When comparing a group of patients with hip osteoarthritis in question for total hip replacement with a group of individuals matched by sex, age and municipality without hip complaints they did not report more co-morbid conditions [3]. Neither did the number of co-morbid conditions predict a non-successful result in WOMAC function at an intermediate follow-up. Except for problems related to the hip, the patients reported a health-related quality of life comparable to the reference group. Musculoskeletal co-morbidities such as low back pain were characteristic of patients with poor outcome in WOMAC function, and preoperative pain was a predictor for a poorer outcome in WOMAC function. The preoperative pain is probably explained by regional pain related to the current hip and in some part to the contralateral hip. Poorer physical function as measured by SF-36 preoperatively was also a predictor of poor outcome in WOMAC function at the intermediate follow-up. These results are to a great extent in agreement with the results of Jones and colleagues [5] and Fortin and colleagues [8].

It has also been demonstrated that the patients with the lowest preoperative scores in function do not reach the same level postoperatively as the patients with the highest preoperative scores [2, 8]. The poor preoperative scores in physical function are certainly a consequence of the impairment of the hip, but may also be influenced by musculoskeletal co-morbidities such as low back pain [9].

12.4
Radiographic Stage of OA

Progression of hip OA in epidemiological studies is often defined by change in joint space narrowing correlated with changes in clinical status [10]. In a previous study from the Department of Orthopaedics at Halmstad Hospital in Sweden, almost all patients had moderate or advanced radiographic OA [11]. Furthermore, the radiographic stage of OA (moderate or severe) did not influence the clinical outcome as measured by SF-36 and WOMAC 1 year postoperatively. Neither was there any relationship between preoperative symptoms and the radiographic stage of OA in established OA. With this knowledge, symptoms and not the degree of radiographic change should provide the indication for surgery, once the diagnosis is established.

12.5
Waiting Time

Previous studies have shown that the waiting time is unrelated to the severity of pain and disability and did not appear to have negative impact on outcome postoperatively [2, 9]. Maybe the current system of prioritising patients does not sufficiently take the patient's own experience of pain and disability into consideration.

12.6
Determinants of Poor Outcome

Hip replacement for OA is above all surgery for relieving pain and improving physical function. Pain relief is experienced very soon after surgery as pointed out before, while the adaptation to the new health-status as expressed by SF-36 (role function) takes at least 1 year [2]. When comparing a group of patients who have received THR with a matched reference group, it is obvious that the patients do not reach the same level of function postoperatively as the reference group.

The determinants for a worse outcome postoperatively when using the level of function as the primary outcome measure seems to be old age, low back pain and pain in the non-operated hip.

The number of co-morbid conditions preoperatively did not predict a worse outcome postoperatively when measured by WOMAC function. The same result was found when using SF-36 PF (physical function) as outcome measure, even though it is expected to show a better gradient with co-morbidities.

Low back pain and pain in the hip *not* operated on is characteristic for patients that do not reach the same level of function postoperatively as the matched reference group. These findings are in concordance with a recently published study [5], and indicate that WOMAC captures not only knee or hip pain and dysfunction but is influenced by the presence of low back pain [12, 13]. The decrease in frequency of reported low back pain after THR observed in the patient cohort could in part be explained by a changed postoperative pain threshold [14], and in part by an improved pain-free range of motion in the operated hip.

The general health status of persons with pain in the hip or knee is comparable to that of a reference group without such pain [15], but the health status is worse when pain in the hip or knee occurs in combination with other mobility restricting conditions, for example pain in other joints and other musculoskeletal problems such as back pain. Pain in the hip not operated on may be a symptom of bilateral OA in these patients [16], even in the absence of radiological change.

The difference in function is explained at least in some part by the presence of musculoskeletal co-morbidities such as low back pain and pain in the non-operated hip. The majority of patients experience a significant improvement in pain and function after THR. However, at 3.6 years after surgery, almost one-third of the patients report only a low degree of improvement or have become worse following the THR. Part of this lack of response may be explained by old age and a high degree of pain at the time of surgery. This is supported by previous reports that have suggested surgery earlier rather than later in the course of OA [17]. A report of low back pain has a significant impact on postoperative function after THR, of importance when planning rehabilitation.

A major proportion of the variability in outcome after THR remains unexplained. Further patient-relevant outcome data collected by the use of self-administered questionnaires, and a better understanding of the role of expectations and satisfaction, is essential to improve our understanding of who does or does not benefit from these surgical procedures. Much effort is focussed on the "technical" aspects of this intervention to further improve its success rate. Perhaps we may stand to gain as much or more outcome improvement by better understanding of these "other" factors.

References

1. MacWilliam CH, Yood MU, Verner JJ, McCarthy BD, Ward RE. Patient-related risk factors that predict poor outcome after total hip replacement. Health Serv Res 1996;31:623–38
2. Nilsdotter AK, Lohmander LS. Age and waiting time as predictors of outcome after total hip replacement for osteoarthritis. Rheumatology (Oxford) 2002;41:1261–7
3. Nilsdotter AK. Patient Relevant Outcome after Total Hip Replacement in Osteoarthritis [bibliography]. Lund: Lund University; 2001
4. Söderman P, Malchau H, Herberts P, Zugner R, Regner H, Garellick G. Outcome after total hip arthroplasty: Part II. Disease-specific follow-up and the Swedish National Total Hip Arthroplasty Register. Acta Orthop Scand 2001;72:113–9
5. Jones CA, Voaklander DC, Johnston DW, Suarez-Almazor ME. The effect of age on pain, function, and quality of life after total hip and knee arthroplasty. Arch Intern Med 2001;161: 454–60
6. Young NL, Cheah D, Waddell JP, Wright JG. Patient characteristics that affect the outcome of total hip arthroplasty: a review. Can J Surg 1998;41:188–95
7. Katz JN, Wright EA, Guadagnoli E, Liang MH, Karlsson EW, Cleary PD. Differences between men and women undergoing major orthopedic surgery for degenerative arthritis. Arthritis Rheum 1994;37:687–94
8. Fortin PR, Penrod JR, Clarke AE, St-Pierre Y, Joseph L, Belisle P, et al. Timing of total joint replacement affects clinical outcomes among patients with osteoarthritis of the hip or knee. Arthritis Rheum 2002;46:3327–30
9. Jones CA, Voaklander DC, Johnston DW, Suarez-Almazor ME. Health related quality of life outcomes after total hip and knee arthroplasties in a community based population. J Rheumatol 2000;27:1745–52
10. Dougados M, Gueguen A, Nguyen M, Berdah L, Lequesne M, Mazieres B, et al. Radiological progression of hip osteoarthritis definition, risk factors and correlations with clinical status. Ann Rheum Dis 1996;356–62
11. Nilsdotter AK, Aurell Y, Siosteen AK, Lohmander LS, Roos HP. Radiographic stage of osteoarthritis or sex of the patient does not predict one year outcome after total hip arthroplasty. Ann Rheum Dis 2001;60:228–32

12

12. Wolfe F. Determinants of WOMAC function, pain and stiffness scores: evidence for the role of low back pain, symptom counts, fatigue and depression in osteoarthritis, rheumatoid arthritis and fibromyalgia. Rheumatology (Oxford) 1999;38:355–61
13. Harcourt WG, White SH, Jones P. Specificity of the Oxford knee status questionnaire. The effect of disease of the hip or lumbar spine on patients' perception of knee disability. J Bone Joint Surg Br 2001;83:345–7
14. Kosek E, Ordeberg G. Lack of pressure pain modulation by heterotopic noxious conditioning stimulation in patients with painful osteoarthritis before, but not following, surgical pain relief. Pain 2000;88:69–78
15. Hopman-Rock M, Odding E, Hofman A, Kraaimaat FW, Bijlsma JW. Differences in health status of older adults with pain in the hip or knee only and with additional mobility restricting conditions. J Rheumatol 1997;24:2416–23
16. Birrell F, Croft P, Cooper C, Hosie G, Macfarlane G, Silman A. Health impact of pain in the hip region with and without radiographic evidence of osteoarthritis: a study of new attenders to primary care. The PCR Hip Study Group. Ann Rheum Dis 2000;59:857–63
17. Fortin P, Clarke A, Joseph L, Liang M, Tanzer M, Ferland D, et al. Outcomes of total hip and knee replacement. Arthritis Rheum 1999;42:1722–8

Evaluation of the Implant

13

Different Perspectives of Outcome Measurement:
Radiography and Alternatives

M. Krismer

13.1
Introduction

Outcome of artificial hip replacement is often perceived as either implant survival or as the subjective judgement of the patient on pain and function. Both parameters address the ideal result of hip arthroplasty, a long-lasting, pain-free hip with good function.

The ideal result cannot be achieved in all cases, and attempts to ameliorate the results will be undertaken in the future. Progress can be expected either by an error and trial approach or by understanding the underlying mechanisms of failure, establishing a model of causes, factors and effects. This may be the main purpose of radiographic methods in *science*.

Radiography also has the goal to give a clue, why the *individual patient* is symptomatic, or will be symptomatic in the future, and will provide some insight in the underlying causes of problems with hip arthroplasty in a particular patient.

X-rays also provide an information on the quality of implantation, whether the surgeon has successfully achieved an optimal implant position, equal leg length and offset. In this sense, X-rays establish a *feedback system for the surgeon* increasing implantation quality.

Radiography is used:

- To determine whether an implant is loose
- To assess category and extension of bone destruction
- To assess bony ingrowth
- To get insight in stress transmission and stress-shielding
- To assess the presence of ossifications
- To assess the implant position
- To assess the amount of polyethylene wear
- To measure migration, the movement of an implant of its bony bed

M. Krismer (✉)
Universitätsklinik für Orthopädie, Anichstrasse 35, 6020 Innsbruck, Austria
e-mail: martin.krismer@uki.at

K.E. Dreinhöfer et al. (eds.), *EUROHIP: Health Technology Assessment of Hip Arthroplasty in Europe*, DOI: 10.1007/978-3-540-74137-4_13, © 2009 EFORT

13.2
Radiographic Assessment of Loosening

Radiolucent lines around the implant are the radiographic representation of fibrous tissue around the implant. There is a general agreement that an implant completely surrounded by fibrous tissue is loose. A loose implant usually migrates, with cups migrating craniad and stems migrating caudad. In both components, the acetabular and the femoral, migration may diminish the thickness of a fibrous tissue layer, and a radiolucent line can completely disappear in one or two zones. Therefore, the radiographic definition of loosening based on an implant completely surrounded by radiolucent lines will be very specific (an implant completely surrounded by radiolucent lines is really loose), but not sensitive enough (an implant not completely surrounded by radiolucent lines may be loose) [1–3].

Radiolucent lines may be caused either by polyethylene wear or by motion of an implant fixed at the end and moving at the other end (cantilever bending mechanism in stems). Therefore, an implant incompletely surrounded by radiolucencies is not always loose.

In keeping with the above mentioned reasons, we can expect to encounter many borderline cases. The assessment of loosening cannot be based on radiolucencies alone. Migration measurement can partially solve the problem, as a migrating implant must considered to be loose, although migration in the first year after implantation may also be caused by some migration before settling of the implant followed by a solid bone–implant surface connection [4]. In the stem, an alternative method, the classification of the pedestal, the bony bridge at the tip of the stem, was developed. Some authors believe that the pedestal in the presence of radiolucencies around the area of the tip of the stem signifies instability. Other authors also point out that the pedestal cannot be interpreted without additional information on migration [3].

13.3
Stress Shielding

The elasticity of bone is far higher than the elasticity of implants, with the rare exception of an isoelastic polyethylene implant. The longer an implant the more is it unlikely that the entire length of the implant is strongly fixed to its bony bed. In cemented implants, the bone cement allows for some micromotion of the implant, and the relatively isoelastic bone cement transmits the stress to the bone, which is always separated from the bone cement by a very thin layer of fibrous tissue. However, in an uncemented stem, stress cannot be equally transmitted from the implant to the bony implant bed. In the case of proximal stress transmission to the stem, the entire femoral bone is loaded, and this will cause no problem. In distal fixation, proximal bone will become osteoporotic due to inactivity. After a couple of years, this can be easily seen in X-rays with thickened cortical bone at the tip of the prosthesis and proximal bone loss. Bone densitometry is more specific than are X-rays for this purpose, and will provide information much earlier.

13.4
Assessment of Bony Ingrowth

In good radiographs, single trabeculae of bone can be seen. The presence of well-developed and thick trabecular bone originating from the surface of an implant, and connecting the surface with the cortical bone of the femur or the cancellous bone of the pelvis, was believed to indicate bony ingrowth. It was often seen in migration studies that implants showing this sign of bony ingrowth had migrated and showed further migration. Therefore, the significance of bony ingrowth in X-rays is low.

13.5
Radiographic Assessment of Bone Destruction

Implant-related osteolysis is usually caused by polyethylene wear, but may also be caused by metal corrosion, infection and perhaps, in rare cases, by an immunologic response to components of cement or the metal alloy. In any case, there is no method to get radiographic insight into the nature of the osteolysis. The extension of bone destruction can be determined on X-rays under the condition that enough bone is destroyed, and that bone destruction is not hidden by the implant. It was shown especially for metastatic disease that only a proportion of osteolysis will be visible, and that CT is much more sensitive for detection of osteolysis. Several classification systems exist in order to give guidelines for revision surgery [5].

Progressive bone destruction can occur in relatively asymptomatic patients and may then establish sufficient reason to propose revision in an otherwise healthy patient without pain, in order to avoid more damage and destruction of bone which will deteriorate the conditions for revision surgery.

13.6
Heterotopic Ossifications

Ossification may be a self-limited and irrelevant finding in X-rays. Frequently, some ossifications occur in the remnants of old haematomas. In some cases, however, muscles around the hip ossify in an inflammatory process, beginning on the day of surgery, and in a painful process leading to severe limitation of hip motion, or even to complete ankylosis due to a bony bridge between the pelvis and the femur. In X-rays, heterotopic ossifications, especially the relevant ones, can be seen and classified [6].

In severe cases, surgery is sometimes required to remove the ossifications to allow for enough hip motion. Then, CT-scans are required to get more information on the extension of ossification.

13.7
Implant Position

In acetabular components, the intented orientation in relation to the pelvis cannot be determined exactly in radiographs [7]. This is due to the fact that the anatomic pelvis plane defined by the anterior superior iliac spines and the pubic tubercles is usually not parallel to the film plane, and that the central beam is centred to the symphysis pubis, so that the projection of the acetabular component depends on an oblique cone geometry, focus-object and focus-film distance, the position of the patient and the position of the central beam. Simple CT-scans cannot overcome this problem. However, coordinates can be determined in CT-scans and can be used to calculate cup position. Alternatively, more sophisticated methods based on X-rays can be used with acceptable accuracy [8]. Traditionally, cup inclination and anteversion is measured. However, several definitions of these parameters exist [9].

In the stem, offset and leg length can be measured in plain X-rays or standing X-rays of the entire leg. Stem rotation cannot be measured in X-rays, but very well in CT-scans, where stem rotation can be related to the posterior condylar line or to the transepicondylar line. Varus–valgus position of the stem axis in relation to the femoral axis is a further stem position parameter.

13.8
Migration Measurement

The migration of an implant in relation to the surrounding bone can be measured best with roentgen stereophotogrammetric analysis (RSA) [10]. This method requires X-rays in a special frame with reference points and simultaneous exposition of two films in defined positions to each other. Repeated expositions over 2 or more years allow for calculation of a curve migration against time (Fig. 13.1). Accuracy is excellent, and is estimated to be far below 1 mm. The error is much higher in plain X-rays, especially due to changing position of pelvis and femur in consecutive radiographs, and amounts to 3 or 5 mm. EBRA is a method based on plain X-rays with an accuracy of about 1 mm, enough for prediction of loosening and revision [4, 8].

Migration is assumed to signify a loose implant. Especially in the first year after implantation, settling and consecutive stabilisation can occur, particularly in uncemented implants. Some cemented implants, especially the Exeter design, are intended to migrate in the cement mantle. Only migration of the cement mantle against the surrounding bone can then be taken as a sign of loosening.

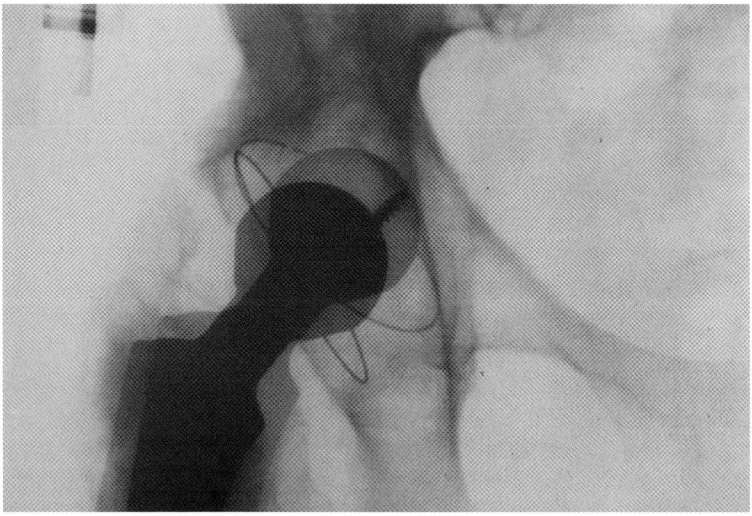

Fig. 13.1 Cup migration: migration of a polyethylene cup and a marker wire in the course of 9 years, where two X-rays showed an almost identical pelvic contour

References

1. DeLee JG, Charnley J (1976) Radiological demarcation of cemented sockets in total hip replacement. Clin Orthop 121:20–4
2. Gruen TA, McNeice GM, Amstutz HC (1979) "Modes of failure" of cemented stem-type femoral components. A radiographic analysis of loosening. Clin Orthop 141:17–27
3. Engh CA, Massin P, Suthers KE (1990) Roentgenographic assessment of the biologic fixation of porous-surfaced femoral components. Clin Orthop 257:107–28
4. Krismer M, Biedermann R, Stöckl B, Fischer M, Bauer R, Haid Ch (1999) The prediction of failure of the stem in THR by measurement of early migration using EBRA-FCA. J Bone Joint Surg 81-B:273–80
5. Paprovsky WG, Burnett RS (2002) Assessment and classification of bone stock deficiency in revision total hip arthroplasty. Am J Orthop 31:459–64
6. Brooker AF, Bowerman JW, Robinson RA, Riley LH Jr (1973) Ectopic ossification following total hip replacement. Incidence and a method of classification. J Bone Joint Surg 55-A:1629–32
7. Lewinnek GE, Lewis JL, Tarr R, Compere CL, Zimmerman JR (1978) Dislocations after total hip-replacement arthroplasties. J Bone Joint Surg 60-A:217–20
8. Krismer M, Bauer R, Tschupik JP, Mayrhofer P (1995) EBRA: a method to measure migration of acetabular components. J Biomech 28:1225–36
9. Murray DW (1993) The definition and measurement of acetabular orientation. J Bone Joint Surg 75-B:228–32
10. Nistor L, Blaha JD, Kjellstrom U, Selvik G (1991) In vivo measurements of relative motion between an uncemented femoral total hip component and the femur by roentgen stereophotogrammetric analysis. Clin Orthop 269:220–7

Result Analysis of Hip Arthroplasty Registers

14

U. Schütz and K. Dreinhöfer

14.1
National Hip Arthroplasty Registers and Their Objective

In the Scandinavian countries Sweden, Norway and Finland, we find the oldest nationwide arthroplasty registers (ARs). Sweden established the first National Hip Arthroplasty Register (NHAR) worldwide in 1979. The mission of the first national hip AR, the Swedish NHAR, was to improve the outcome of total hip arthroplasty (THA) [30]. Throughout the 1970s, new hip implants had been introduced without documentation from clinical studies. After being used for more than 10 years, several of the prostheses were identified with high failure rates, but at the time they had already been used in large numbers of patients. Intending to identify inferior implants as soon as possible, several more countries have started national ARs in the last 15 years. Initiated by their national orthopaedic associations, Finland (1980) and Norway (1987) both started during the 1980s, and the Danish Hip Arthroplasty Register (DHAR) [41] followed in 1994. In the larger European States with 50-80 million inhabitants (United Kingdom, France, Germany, Italy, Spain), national registers have not so far been established. Outside Europe, national registers were established later. Following a pilot study in 1997 in Christchurch, a national joint register was established by the New Zealand Orthopaedic Association in January 2000. In March 1998, the Federal Government provided funding to the Australian Orthopaedic Association (AOA) to establish the National Joint Replacement Registry (NJRR). The Canadian Joint Replacement Registry (CJRR) was officially launched at the Canadian Orthopaedic Association annual meeting in June 2000 and is managed by the Canadian Institute for Health Information (CIHI). Even the USA now finds that the time has come for a national joint replacement register, and planning for pilot projects for implementation has begun [46] (Table 14.1).

An AR should serve the quality assurance in joint replacement surgery. The main purpose of an AR is to identify existing differences in regional or national joint replacement

U. Schütz (✉)
Department of Orthopedics, Ulm University, Oberer Eselsberg 45, 89081 Ulm, Germany
e-mail: uwe.schuetz@uniklinik-ulm.de;karsten.dreinhoefer@uni-ulm.de

K.E. Dreinhöfer et al. (eds.), *EUROHIP: Health Technology Assessment of Hip Arthroplasty in Europe*, DOI: 10.1007/978-3-540-74137-4_14, © 2009 EFORT

14

Table 14.1 Established arthroplasty registers

AP	Popul. (10^6 n)	Over all (n)	Joint	Reg. start	Doc. reg. end	Reg. period (years)	pTA (n)	rTA (n)	Revisions (%)	LDY	Incidence pTA (n/10^5)	Incidence rTA (n/10^5)	Annual report (AR); literature; sources
Sweden*: NHAR, n	8.9	>350,000	THA	1979	2002	23	252,547	19,620	8.4	2002	157.9	16.4	AR 1998 [45], 2000 [44], 2002 [43]; [32, 60]
SKAR, n[a]	8.9		TKA	1985	2002	17	77,805	4,285	5.5	2002	76.0	–	AR 1999, 2001, 2002, 2003; [54, 55]
Norway (NAR), n	4.5	140,000	THA	1987	2004	17	101,500	14,403	14.2	2003	154.4	21.4	AR 2002, 2003, 2004; [19, 21, 26–28]
			TKA			8	16,080	1,499	9.3		66.8	5.4	
			TSA				1,406	127	9.0		3.9	0.3	
			TEA				494	113	22.9		1.1	0.2	
			TWA	1994	2003		89	10	11.2		0.2	0.0	
			FA				2,770	334	12.1		3.9	0.6	
			TAA				179	32	17.9		0.5	0.2	
			TA				682	128	18.8		1.5	0.4	
Finland* (FER), n[a]	5.2	>75,000	THA	1980	2001	21	74,496	15,172	20.4	2001	107.1	23.5	AR 1998– 1999, 2000– 2001; [53]
			TKA				48,249	4,067	8.4		102.2	7.8	
			TSA				1,919		–		3.9	–	
			TEA				1,429				1.9		
			FA				3,162				3.5		
			TAA				183				1.1		
			TA				183				0.0		
Dänemark* (DHAR), n	5.4	>22,000	THA	1995	1998	4	18,222	3,343	18.3	1998	91.5	–	[32]

Register			Type										Report
New Zealand (NJR), n	4.0	>45,000	THA	1999	2003	5	25,349	3,608	14.2	2003	119.5	17.9	AR 2003; [57]
			TKA	2000	2003	4	17,678	1,128	6.4		84.9	8.7	
			TSA				763	17	2.2		4.8	–	
			TEA				110	16	14.5		0.8	0.2	
			TAA				108	2	1.9		0.7	–	
Australia (NJRR), n	20	>320,000	THA	1998	2002	4	174,764	13,256	7.6	2002	117.5	19.1	AR 2000, 2001, 2002, 2003
			TKA				147,795	8,151	5.5		121.7	11.9	
Canada (CJRR), n[a]	32.5	>310,000	THA	1994	2002	8	148,899		–	2001	57.4	–	AR 2002. 2003. 2004
			TKA		2003	9	161,798				72.4		
Scotland (SAP), r/n	5.0	~100,000	THA	1991	2003	12	47,910	15,925	33.2	2002	86.0	14.4	AR 2002, 2003, 2004
			TKA				31,990	2,519	7.9		69.0	6.0	
UK*, r[b]	60.1	–	THA	1990	1997	7	~1,400	–	–	–	–	–	[4, 15, 16]
UK* (NJR), n[b]	60.1	Records: 100,000	THA	2003	2004	1	–	–	–	–	–	–	
Romania*, n (RAR)	22.4	20,000	THA	2001	2004	3	17,385	1,036	6.0	2002	23.2	1.4	Report 2001–2003
	22.4		TKA	2003		1	1,275	37	2.9		1.9	0.1	
Italy*, r[b,c] (RIPO)	58.2	~26,000	THA	1990	2002	13	~20,000		–	–	–	–	Report 2000–2002
			TKA	1995	2002	7	~6,000						
Germany* (DER) J[a,b]	82.4	~30,000	THA	1997	1999	2	17,766	2,989	16.8	–	–	–	[40, 52]
			TKA				8,336	793	9.5				
Iceland, n[b]	0.3	>5,000	THA	1992	1996	4	3,403	–	–	1996	52	–	[33]
			THA	2003		0	–	–	–				
United States (Medicare)[b]	293	–											AAOS, 1999
			TKA	2003							92		

n National, r regional, l local, pTA primary total arthroplasty, rTA revision total arthroplasty, THA total hip arthroplasty, TKA total knee arthroplasty, TSA total shoulder arthroplasty, TEA total elbow arthroplasty, TWA total wrist arthroplasty, FA finger arthroplasty, TAA total ankle arthroplasty, TA toe arthroplasty

*EU state

[a] Rate includes all total and partial knee replacements

[b] Data is not representative of full population

[c] Includes both primary and revision total arthroplasties

14

results and to identify inferior implants as early as possible [23]. In quality assessment of health technology, procedures like THA structural quality, process quality and result quality must be distinguished [12]. In recent years, health associations, health insurance organisations and state health institutions of many European countries established control and documentation instruments, but usually only taking into account the recording of the structure and process quality. The evaluation of result quality is not possible when the data recording ends at the time of clinical discharge of the patient [13]. But it is the result quality which is the decisive dimension for THA assessment procedures. This dimension can be reached by development of AR with data acquisition containing the complete period of time, from implantation until failure or the end of survival time. To make results objective and comparisons possible, the result quality can be evaluated with standardised criteria [24, 25, 34, 35, 48].

14.2
Structure of Arthroplasty Registers

The opinions regarding the question which organisation or institution should operate an AR differ. In countries with already existing national registers, these are led and organised by the corresponding national orthopaedic society.

The Swedish NHAR consists of three different databases: the primary hip replacement database includes information on the interventions per year and clinic (1979–1991) with registration of the number of operations, type of implant, diagnosis and operated side. The second, the revision database, is derived from analysis of the hospital records from all reoperated patients since 1979. The third is related to the surgical technique and includes information on preventive actions against aseptic loosening. The cementing technique, cement type, prophylactic antibiotics and other preventive data are also reported yearly. The Danish DHAR was organised on about the same principles as the NHAR in Sweden. In the Norwegian NAR, the orthopaedic surgeons provide information from all primary joint replacements, including an accurate description of the different parts of the implant. If the prosthesis is revised later, possibly at a different hospital, it receives a new report with information about the reason for and the type of revision.

In the majority of the cases where national registers work comprehensively and universally, a comparison has always been available or established between register database and municipal or nationwide authority databases. The special linkage key feature for this is an unique individual civic ID-number of every national citizen, which is used not only for public state facilities but also for data pools like an AR. In the Scandinavian countries, the use of a social security number for all inhabitants is unique. In Sweden, this ID-number includes information such as date of birth and gender and is used by everyone in all contacts with authorities, hospitals and most private companies when identification is required. The ID is readily available, is printed on ID-cards and passports, and permits life-long tracing of patients including date of death. For the annual reports of 2002 [43], a linkage of the primary hip replacement database of NHAR to future revisions was necessary, for example, and the unique Swedish ID number was used. For 90% of the clinics, this information is nowadays reported on-line through the internet. In the Norwegian NAR, the revisions are linked to their primary operations by using the patients' national social security numbers. Information on dates of death of deceased patients can be obtained from the Norwegian Population Registry.

Joint replacement data for the Canadian register are obtained from four sources: non-Ontario orthopaedic surgeons participating in the CJRR, Ontario surgeons in the OJRR, and two hospital separation databases managed by the CIHI, the Hospital Morbidity Database and the Discharge Abstract Database (DAD). The DAD provides the number of discharges (including deaths) from a hospital by primary diagnosis and contains all acute care discharges in Canada. The Hospital Morbidity Database contains a number of different clinical and demographic data. The CIHI receives data directly from participating hospitals, which represent about 85% of all hospital inpatient discharges in Canada.

As this survey of data documentation of established national AR shows, there are different possibilities of the structural organisation and the data interchange. These depend much on the underlying conditions and possibilities regarding the political situation, the data protection laws and the financial and technical support as well as the intended objectives. The most vital part for a national AR is to be as precise and comprehensive as possible at the local level. The other part is a good linkage to other national databases.

The described registers are mostly subsidised by the state since through their existence the national budget and, especially, the health budget are considerably relieved. The principle of a register leadership by the responsible national orthopaedic society with financial governmental support works well in countries of a defined size, if the local departments can also recognize an advantage for themselves in a central data registration. The possibility of such a nationwide comprehensive data registration in countries like the size of Germany seems to be unsatisfactory until now. The main difficulties are persuading all orthopaedic departments and surgeons to participate at the register. The solution of these difficulties could be that the payment for an arthroplasty implantation is only carried out to the performing unit when the registration of the treatment is already done. Regarding both implantation process with follow-up treatment and payment, the arthroplasty registration should therefore ideally become a component of the whole procedure. An embedding of the manufacturers in these considerations and structural questions is therefore indispensable. Development of these structures needs political decisions, while corresponding development of informed opinion processes are necessary and, of course, depend very strongly on the respective political and social framework conditions of the specific country. In principle, a national AR should always be led by the responsible national orthopaedic society, while government financial support (the payment of a proportional share of the financial consideration should not be to the clinical complexes but direct to the AR) and close cooperation with the health authorities is necessary. A register can be and should be financed by the state and has to be independent from the medical device industry.

14.3
Requirements on Documentation

An exact, purposeful documentation of data is an essential prerequisite for quality ensuring measures. Comparing the Swedish NHAR with the Norwegian NAR shows that the Norwegians can get much more detailed information from their register. Quality differences

14

exist with the following reasons and essential differences. Sweden has two separate registers for hip and knee APL. They do not distinguish between individual cup and stem components [22]. The register does not collect radiological information [22] nor anything about the quality of life or mortality [59]. The Norwegian NAR is considerably more innovative here. Survival probabilities can be calculated for each of the prosthetic components [26, 27], pain, function and patient satisfaction are documented [27] and complications like infection and dislocation are also noted.

The prospective recording of data using standardised clinical and radiological appraisal factors is the aim of the documentation, which should be partitioned into demographic patient data, peri-operative data, pre- and postoperative data, clinical and radiological follow-up data [13].

14.4
Acceptance, Compliance and Transparency

The acceptance and compliance of an AR in the profession is the limiting factor regarding success and correct data collection. Everybody involved in the information process should profit from a register. The acceptance of quality assurance measures like an AR increases if the immediate results are discussed transparently and with those involved. Quality assurance means the analysis or support of processes and not the denouncing of personal faults. The data analysis should be process- and not person-oriented.

The presentation of the results of the data evaluation should be carried out regularly so that everyone can participate, discuss and decide on necessary consequences. The methods result presentation are varied: presentation of annual reports to participating units, presentation of printed annual surveys, of all data with full lists of input and cumulative revision rates (CRRs); arranging of annual meetings with contact persons, the manufacturers or sales-people; presentation of results at national and international meetings; and publications of papers in peer-reviewed journals, and of selected reports and reference lists on the world wide web.

All orthopaedic departments in Sweden producing THA surgery participate in the Swedish NHAR on a voluntary basis. More than 95% of the total hip operations are reported to the register [61]. Investigations of the Norwegian NAR have shown that at least 95% of all joint replacements performed are reported to the register. In September 2003, 63% of orthopaedic surgeons performing total hip and total knee replacement surgery in Canada were participating in the Canadian CJRR. The compliance for the Romania RAR was 74–84% at the last control. The compliance can be reduced by different reasons, some of which may not be predictable. In the Danish DHAR, the incidence of primary THA (93/100,000 inhabitants, 1995) is presumably too low because of underreporting, indicated by a higher reporting of similar operations from public hospitals to the National Board of Health. The low number of operations may be due to a long hospital strike in that year.

To increase the compliance and acceptance of a national register, some countries go further. In Canada, at the CJRR, participating surgeons can earn Continuing Professional Development (CPD) credits by submitting operative data to the CJRR and reviewing regular CJRR feedback reports. Submission of six completed data collection forms to CIHI will earn each surgeon one credit. The legal obligation to participation would be an opportunity towards an increase in compliance if the acceptance is not sufficient on a voluntary basis.

14.5
Parameters, Items

Before the recording and documentation, the relevant parameters had to be defined. This is just as necessary for comparisons within a register and between different registers than a prerequisite for a uniting of single registers into larger ones. For example, the term "reoperation" can be defined in different ways. The general definition would be: "Every new operation of a patient who has already received a THA in the past". A specification is, however, necessary for the purposes of a register: "Any new operation which is connected with the THA operation the patient underwent before". The Swedish NHAR further specifies: "Any new hip operation on a patient who has previously undergone total hip replacement". The definition of this parameter has a direct influence on the evaluation of relevant outcome-parameters, such as the CRR and the revision burden (RB). These too must, however, be predefined (see Section 14.8 "Outcome key parameters").

However, depending on the analytical question, the definitions can also be newly defined again and again at the statistical processing of the register data. Furthermore, subdividing and grouping is possible when the parameter recording is carried out in detail. For example, in the Swedish NHAR, the definition for revision varied from 2002 to 2004. Global definition: exchange or removal of one or both components. Exchange of liner or head component is considered a revision but also not. Distinction: revision is defined as a *first* exchange of cup, stem or both. Permanent girdlestone procedures, exchange of liner or head component were excluded. Two types of end-points were used: a component specific (i.e. cup or stem re-revision) and a non-component specific (i.e. revision for any reason).

The higher the register level (national, international AR) the more selected and reduced the item variety is compared to the lower level (regional, local AR). Experience from established registers indicates that the demands on the possibilities of differentiated evaluation increases with time and limitation occurs through restricted item recording. If linkage to other databases or additional data transmission is not possible, certain evaluations are then not feasible.

14.6
Evaluation of Factors Influencing Survival of THA

Insufficient outcome data and the variability of results focussing on specific diagnosis-, patient-, implant-, surgical method-related factors and characteristics, which can influence the success, have made it difficult for the surgeons to identify the relative effectiveness of the different prostheses and treatments. The specific functions of an AR are to describe the epidemiology of joint replacement surgery and to identify factors associated with an increased risk for revision and inferior outcome. Reducing or changing of all the factors,

14

which were recognized as negative influence factors on the revision rate, must lead to an improvement on the result quality.

The demographic factor. The main patient-related factor, age, is the outstanding epidemiological demographic factor for future decades because the main indication for THA is the age-related disease OA. Previously, joint replacement was reserved for the elderly. However, due to the success of the procedure it is increasingly used in younger individuals. This, combined with an aging population, has resulted in an increase of incidence of primary THA in all countries performing this operation. The rate of total revision hip arthroplasty (TRHA) is also increasing. More patients are living longer than the life expectancy of the joint replacement. Revision surgery is associated with increased morbidity and mortality and has a far less successful outcome than primary joint replacement. As such, it is essential to ensure that everything possible is done to limit the rate of revision surgery.

Indication and priorisation finding. The USA are performing the most THA in absolute terms but have a lower incidence than most European countries; there must be differences in indications and prioritisation. Countries with an existing hip AR are able to give exact data about the incidence progression for THA and TRHA. The data from countries without such a register came from different sources. For example, regarding the national absolute THA number per year in Germany, the comparison of data from manufacturers with public sources like registers and hospitals differ. There were more prostheses sold than are documented as implanted (Fig. 14.1). The data are not directly comparable. Depending on the data source, very different details which often show considerable discrepancies are available. To receive exact data regarding the prosthetic quality and number, an AR is necessary.

Technical data. Besides the indication finding process, the choice of the implantation method also plays an essential role. The choice of the technical procedure depends on patient-related factors, but essentially on the implant-related factors and possibilities.

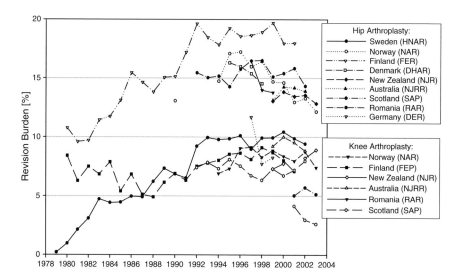

Fig. 14.1   Annual number primary THA in OECD-countries. Data for graph with special permission from [49]

Regarding selection criteria for a specific implantation procedure of THA, the following parameters are relevant: implantation technique, procedures (fixation technique, surgical approach), implants (cup, inlay, head, stem), cement types, tribology, component sizes, material processing (surface, design) and surgical experience.

The implant factor. As a product of new technologies, there are an increasing number and variety of prostheses that are available on the (inter-)national markets. For many of these, the mid- to long-term survival rates remain unknown. For a register, it is easy to document the component characteristics of implanted THAs. The only need is for information about the producer (manufacturing company) and the product ID-number with labelling. Having these data, the following data are incorporated for every component: material, design, surface, modularity and size. This exact description of the implant components used by product-ID-number will facilitate analysis of implant properties. Importance has to be given in documenting the component combination forming a THA, by giving information about tribology.

Health and self assessment scores. In recent years, the study of other types of outcome measures, not based on failures, such as patient satisfaction, general and disease-specific health scores, began. Thus, in most patients who do not experience failure, grading of the success may be possible, further enhancing the choice of implants and methods maximally benefitting patients. For the New Zealand Joint Register, approximately 6 months after surgery all registered patients are sent a questionnaire to measure the outcome of their surgery. This can now be answered on-line. The combination of technical data about the joint implanted and the individual patient assessment will give valuable information for New Zealand-based research. However, in most registers, quality of life and subjective satisfaction remains unconsidered at the control examinations although this is the dominating factor in the patient's mind. For interpretation of quality of life in THA, the inclusion of specially developed "Health assessment Scores" (SF-36 [8], WOMAC [2, 3, 62, 63], etc.) is required. However, a uniform opinion on applicability of this scores in the field of hip arthroplasty does not yet exist. Some scores seem to deliver better validity and reliability in this area (e.g. EuroQual [18], subjective health rating scale).

Clinical data. Unlike this, the parameters which had to be registered for evaluation of the accepted objective hip scores (HHS [25], MD [47, 48], etc.) succeeded for the description of the clinical follow-up. A register therefore documents the parameters pain, ADL, function and ROM.

Radiographic data. A pilot project has been initiated in the Western Region of Sweden including approximately 2,000 THA annually. This project collects prospectively a generic health score and subjective satisfaction for all patients as well as radiographic information. This enables early detection of clinically silent osteolysis and loosening. In a future perspective, this gives a possibility to apply cost-utility analyses and consequently tools for an optimal resource allocation in the health care sector. Evaluation will show if this type of data collection is possible and feasible.

Digital migration analysis, early failure detection. Clinical examinations alone are not sensitive enough to detect early loosening [9], and symptoms may appear years after early radiographic changes. Apart from periprosthetic bone reactions [7, 24, 35], the migration of THA-components is the cardinal radiographic sign for loosening. Several independent studies show that a subsidence of the stem of more than 1-2 mm within 2 years after implantation is correlated with a significantly higher probability of implant failure in later years [5, 36, 64]. If migration of a cup is shown, this implant has failed. The digital biplanar migration analysis has reached a high standard regarding precision and predictive value. Some measuring systems can already be downloaded via the world wide web (EBRA [6, 37-39], UMA [5, 10, 11, 29], DMA [50, 51, 58]). Unfortunately, these methods are not being sufficiently used and are not yet included in the THA follow-up procedures of the most clinics. In the near future, these methods will become indispensable for quality assurance of implants, because of the necessity of an early detection of failures will increase and is being demanded.

Surgical experience. Several studies have shown that the experience of the surgeon is also a relevant factor influencing the survival rate and quality of a THA [14, 17]. But this parameter is not documented in any register directly, until now. Reasons for this may be obvious and mostly understandable, but as tendencies in several countries show, experience may become a relevant criteria in the near future. Consideration if being given to couple the permission for THA operations with a minimal number being performed in a particular unit. As alarming as this may be for departments with low case numbers, a limitation of performance suppliers will improve the quality of THA.

14.7
Result Processing

Statistics. It must be kept in mind that these register-based studies are observational. Still, results from register-based studies are less conclusive than those of comparable randomised trials. Regarding the statistical tests, initially the Wilcoxon, the log-rank and other similar tests were used by the Scandinavian registers to test crude (empirical) survival between groups. However, these methods have the disadvantage that, when comparing groups (i.e. implant type), the effect of other factors (i.e. age, gender) is not taken into account. Therefore, in recent years, multiple regression (e.g. Cox model) has been chosen to estimate differences in survival, allowing adjustment for external factors. Due to the immense data size, the multi-factoriality and the importance of a statistically correct evidence-based evaluation and result finding of registered data, statistical analysis has to be done by professional experts such as bio-mathematicians and statisticians. The existing national registers already delegate these activities to appropriate institutions.

Result presentation. Depending on their size and structure, national ARs are able to make extensive epidemiological result analyses and to present them openly in tabular and graphical form. The most important outcome presentations are averages, distributions and developments (changes, prognosis) of age, gender, diagnoses, operative parameters, revisions and complications. The analysis can be focussed on different periods of time (every year, per decade, etc.). Comparative analyses (differences, dependencies) related to particular other parameters (subgroups, cohorts) are possible.

Depending on the statistical methods and parameters used, outcome analysis can be presented very differently on the same topic. A uniform agreement should be found to ensure comparability between the registers. Regarding this, outcome key parameters are already defined in established registers, but their presentation is still carried out differently.

14.8
Outcome Key Parameters

Incidence, prevalence. Prevalence is an important epidemiological parameter for charac-
terisation of the frequency of a certain expression in an examined population; it is always
evaluable from the registered data. The incidence, as a measure for the representation of
the new appearance of a certain expression within a defined time period, refers to the complete population. Only well-functioning registers can give details on incidence regarding
the main diagnoses (e.g. OA, aseptic loosening) or hip arthroplasties (THA, TRHA) of a
country. It is mostly presented as number per 100,000 inhabitants.

Revision = endpoint of failure? Although commonly used, the terms success and failure
were difficult to define in the context of surgical intervention, where the primary objectives
of a treatment can be different. Even apparent obvious failures (e.g. loosening, instability,
wear) are not easily distinguishable from normal postoperative conditions. In view of the
work with clinical follow-up examinations and lack of definitions for all types of failure,
other simpler means became used as indicators of failure. An additional operation, a revision, therefore indicated that both the patient and surgeon agreed that the original problem
has not been solved, so that a revision meant a failure of the primary operation.

In the Swedish NHAR, the endpoint for failure is revision. Three categories of reoperations can be analysed: revision with change or extraction of a prosthetic component, major
reoperation, and minor surgical procedure. In the Swedish NHAR, revision is the predomi-
nant procedure, accounting for approx. 85% of reoperations with major surgical procedures making up about 10% and minor procedures approx. 5% [60].

A prosthesis still in place, however, does not mean success. Soderman et al. [60] performed a clinical outcome analysis on patients with primary total hip replacement thus
testing the adequacy of the endpoint for failure in the NHAR.

A total of 1,113 randomly selected patients who had had THA between 1986 and 1995
answered the disease-specific, self-administered WOMAC questionnaire [2, 3]. A cohort
of 344 patients was studied, using the HHS [25] and a conventional radiographic examination as outcome measures. They found clinical failure rates of 13% and 20% for all implants
after 10 years, using 60 points or revision as the definition of failure in the HHS and
WOMAC, respectively. The result, according to the register during the same period, was a
7% revision rate. The radiological failure rate was evaluated with 9%, using a radiolu-
cency >2 mm in more than two zones as the definition for failure. The clinical failure rate
depended on the type of evaluation tool, definition of failure and demographics, which
made it difficult to decide whether there was a need for revision. With the exception of
pain measured by the HHS, the results showed no significant correlation between clinical
failure and radiographic failure.

With the knowledge that there is a difference between the revision rate according to the
register and clinical outcome, a strict definition of revision in the register is useful as an
endpoint for primary THA. The failure endpoint currently used, revision, is clear and
precise but, as demonstrated, limited. The quality of THA is evaluated based on the survival time of the prostheses, where survival time is defined as the time period from inser-
tion of the prosthesis to its revision. A premature termination of follow-up (so-called

14

censored observations) will be registered if the study is closed, or the patient dies or emigrates with the prosthesis still intact. The outcome presentation of revision can be done differently: survival analysis with the classic Kaplan–Meier curve, with 95% CI (e.g. in the reports of FER, NAR, DHAR) or multivariate Cox regression models.

Cumulative revision rate. The first reports from the Swedish NHAR were mainly descriptive where the number of complications or failures was related to the number of implants. The problem with this simple method was that the operations were not performed all at once and were followed for a different number of years. This, combined with the death of some patients, resulted in patients having different lengths of follow-up, which could produce misleading results. Therefore, survival analyses of data can be shown in graphical curves presenting the CRR as the frequency of revision. The CRR describes what percentage of the operated patients became revised with time. The calculation is based on the sum of all the revisions and expresses the rate as if none of the patients had died. It can be demonstrated in different forms analysing other parameters (implant type, fixation technique, gender, regions, local units, surgical experience, diagnosis, perioperative care, environmental profile and more).

Revision burden. Malchau et al. [43] recommend the introduction of the general outcome parameter "RB". RB is a permanent parameter in the Swedish NHAR annual reports [44, 45]. This parameter should in future be indicated in all registers to ensure their comparability. RB is the fraction of revisions and the total number of primary and revision joint replacement. A wide variation is noted in RB depending on different implant fixation techniques, implant factors and pre-operations. As they are determinable from the annual reports or other sources, the register-based RB of hip and knee arthroplasties from different nations in the period from 1995 to 2003 are shown in Table 14.2 and Fig. 14.2.

Table 14.2 Register based RB

Register; source	Time period	HA	KA
Sweden* (NHAR), n	1995–2002	9.8	– (CRR)
Norway (NAR), n	1995–2003	14.9	8.4
Finland* (FER), n[a]	1995–2001	18.7	8.3
Denmark* (DHAR), n	1995–1998	15.6	–
New Zealand (NJR), n	1999–2003	13.4	8.0
Australia (NJRR), n	1999–2002	13.9	9.4
Scotland (SAP), r/n	1995–2002	15.5	7.2
Romania* (RAR), n	2001–2003	5.3	3.2
Germany* (DER), [a,b]	1997–1999	14.7	9.2
England [43]	2000	15	–
United States (Medicare)[b] [43]	1998	18	–

n National, *r* regional, *l* local, – not available, *HA* hip arthroplasty, *KA* knee arthroplasty, *CRR* cumulative revision rate

*EU state

[a] Rate includes all total and partial knee replacements

[b] Data is not representative of full population: medicare population (older than 65 years)

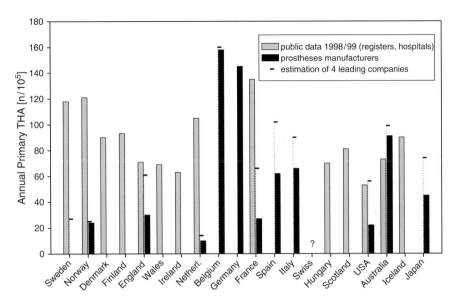

Fig. 14.2   Revision burden of hip and knee arthroplasties based on national register information

14.9
Comparison and Linkage of Registers

In order to facilitate comparisons between different national registries, identification of "key parameters" is important. RB is an example of such a parameter. Tendencies can be seen towards the linkage of existing registers. In April 2003, a national joint registry was launched in England and Wales. The aim of this registry is to collect data pertaining to hip and knee replacements, including detailed information about the types of prosthetic joint implants used. At present, the Scottish Arthroplasty Project (SAP) does not collect these data, but ultimately the Scottish data will be added to the English and Welsh data. In North America the flow of Ontario Joint Replacement Register (OJRR) data to the Canadian CJRR via the Ontario Ministry of Health and Long-Term Care is a landmark event in the history of the CJRR. Ontario is estimated to have one-third (34%) of orthopaedic surgeons in Canada who perform hip and knee replacements. With over 7,500 additional procedures from the OJRR, Ontario data now comprise almost half (45%) of the CJRR 2002-2003 dataset.

14.10
Benefits and Advantages of AR

The Scandinavian countries with national ARs have shown in their annual reports which information, benefits and advantages can be expected from the result finding and statistical evaluation in the long run. These registers has proved their usefulness in many ways beyond the scope of this article and only some general examples will be given.

14

Research benefits. Outcome analyses are the main purpose of an AR when starting. Due to the low failure rate, especially on subsets of patients or implants, further studies can be based only on large multi-centre studies like AR. Large numbers are often needed to detect changes in trends, as well as regional variations in procedures and treatment specifities. Additionally, a large sample size is necessary to carry out meaningful analyses of associations and predictions. The established Scandinavian registers have up to now mainly had a good look at the revision rate and most scientific refurbishing was concentrated on it.

Identification of *risk factors* regarding the failures of THA leading to revision procedures is vital. An example from the Norwegian NAR can be given. A Cox regression analysis from Havelin et al. [27] with adjustment for antibiotic in cement, age, and gender showed that femoral components implanted with the low viscosity cement CMW3 ($n = 1,196$; RR = 2.4, $p < 0.0001$) or the Boneloc cement ($n = 764$; RR = 8.7, $p < 0.0001$) had an increased risk of revision due to aseptic loosening compared to high viscosity cemented implants ($n = 3,788$). Both cements were abandoned in Norway.

Identification of risk factors for failure in TRHA that influence the *re-revision rate* of specific patient populations and of implant-related factors gives the possibility of better standard procedures regarding the indication-finding process and the technical approach to TRHA. At present, there is scant scientific evidence regarding which method is to be used with respect to age, functional demands, bone loss and life expectancy. Many current revision techniques are not evidence-based, and much of the literature originates from the inventors or other centres of excellence. Thus, there is a high risk of performance bias. Interpretation of results depend on the surgeon, long-term national results being so far unknown. Again, the Swedes, with their NHAR [43], are the front runners. Using re-revision of any site as the endpoint, an important finding was that the early first revision dramatically increased the risk of a re-revision. A multivariate patient- and implant-related risk model description is possible.

Epidemiological and demographical analyses are obvious needs for a national AR, and are often included in reports, evaluation reporting and updates of national and regional epidemiological surveys of THA. Due to the rising prevalences regarding implantation, an update regarding indication-finding processes in THA and TRHA in defined time intervals is a main part of the work of a national AR. This should evaluate and influence changes regarding the implants, the fixation techniques and operative technical innovations. Spin-off research projects based on the registers have proved valuable.

Quality benefits. Surgeons could be warned of inferior implants, technically demanding implants, and diseases not to be treated with certain methods and treatments. The AR has the potential to bring problems to attention long before they would be reported and accepted by traditional clinical research methods.

Detection of trends are important regarding the specialisation of different clinics or types of clinics and their establishment of new technologies as quality assurance tools. In Sweden, for example, a decrease in procedure frequency for all types of primary THA is noted for university hospitals. This trend is worrying as most of the clinical research is performed at the tertiary hospitals in Sweden. The surgeons in Sweden have supported the concept of stepwise introduction. This implies that new technology is documented in randomised trials, often by use of RSA prior to widespread clinical use. A further activity reduction at university hospitals will reduce clinical research, and therefore potentially imply a negative effect on the outcome of THA in Sweden. The increase in frequency of THA in rural hospitals indicates, however, that the standard procedure can be performed with good results even in small units.

By collecting individual results of local units, general failure rates and demographic data, comparisons can be made between units and between implants regarding both patient selection and availability of surgery. This helps decision-making and increases the probability of suitable choices. Further, it reveals differences, between regions or patient groups, regarding results and availability or type of treatment being offered. Regional, national and international comparison and matching of different registers and databases multiply the information profit, since further connections can be recognized. Thus, inter-register analyses will give further information about special questions which may be of interest to and motivated by other groups like health politicians or by someone else. The data comparison can also give further information for the register to fill missing values. The Swedish NHAR was therefore matched with the Swedish Death Register. Marked differences in RB are already observed between different countries today (Fig. 14.2).

As a result of detecting dependences between factors in THA, the register gives the possibility of providing prognostic and predictive values regarding specific issues. Indirect information profit about the quality of medical therapies in other areas are also possible. An example may be the decrease of THA surgery in inflammatory arthritis in the Swedish NHAR, which could reflect the improved outcome of modern drug treatment for rheumatoid arthritis [43].

Motivation. ARs can and must be able in the future to promote and to satisfy the motivations for quality assurance in THA. There are different motives for the execution of quality assurance. With regard to generally ethical motives, every person should have the right to the best possible health supply. In the health service, the employees must be interested in working to a high quality standard (professional ethics) and, with increasingly more competent patients, the patient-oriented processes should be advanced. The protection of the patient has to have highest priority (security motives). A higher efficiency should contrast with increasing costs in the health service (efficiency motives) and the participants wanting to receive information about their own performance (performance motive). Learning from their own faults and critical interpretation of their own actions by analysing their own transparent data can lead the participant to quality self-improvement regarding quality (self-educational motives).

Data obtained by registers may encourage the individual departments and individual surgeons to do their best. When hospitals compare their results to those reported nationally, those with inferior results should be stimulated to analyse the reasons and to improve, while others with good results should be motivated to stay at the top. The hypothesis for the project of Sweden's NHAR was that feedback of analysed data stimulates the individual clinic to reflect and improve according to the principle of the good example. The development of the RB in this country in comparison to others seems to prove them right. Having access to nationwide results, surgeons are stimulated to select well-documented methods and implant types.

Benefits of advice. Due to its comprehensive summary, a register is able to show the state of the art of a region or nation in THA. It can describe the current practices in THA, providing accurate information on the use of different types of prostheses in both primary and revision joint replacements. It is regarded as the most effective method of determining which implants and surgical techniques are most successful for given demographic and diagnostic sub-groups. The AR therefore represents a decisive evidence-based epidemiological tool. Surgeons and institutions participating in the registry will receive regular feedback and comparative reports and analyses. Patients are also being guided when information from the register is used to explain what they can expect (risk evaluation), why specific methods are preferred and when to wait or proceed with surgery.

Benefits for the profession. Purchasers of medical treatment, authorities or clients are more willing to give financial support when effects of previous financing can be shown, the results of the treatment can be documented, improvement in quality with time can be demonstrated and future trends can be predicted. ARs can provide this information which helps the orthopaedic profession in the struggle for meagre medical resources.

Benefits for the health care system. Information from ARs will aid in the development of evidence-based practice and guidelines for total replacement surgeries. The application of such evidence-based guidelines improves the results of these operative methods by a reduction of the accompanying morbidities and is therefore leading to systematic general cost savings. The results of the established Scandinavian AR indicate which immense secondary costs the ignoring of influence factors on arthroplasty failure and nationwide uncontrolled and unregistered THA can arise. However, they also show which saving potential an internal, national and international registration of THA can produce according to an adequate quality assurance.

Economic impact. In Sweden, the clinical and socio-economic effects of the past 20 years of NHAR work have been striking. The NHAR has defined the epidemiology of THA in Sweden [42, 43] and the number of hip implants has gone down dramatically. As a result of the register, six implants constitute 70% of the hip market in Sweden. The revision rate (referring to the lifetime of patient) is going down too: from 18% at the start to 6.8% in 1999 (9- to 10-year survival rate: 93-98.3%). The age at time of revision is rising steadily. The range in quality between the different departments is getting smaller, indicating a standardisation on higher levels.

Regarding these points and comparing the RB between different countries (in 1998, the RB in Sweden was 10%, in the United States 18%; see Table 14.2), the Swedish NHAR has had a major economic influence on the national health care costs. Malchau et al. indicate the cost of their NHAR with approximately US$400,000 per year, nearly US$4.00 per registered case and year. The cost for one TRHA is nearly US$12,000. So they conclude that a cost-effectiveness of the NHAR if the annual number of revisions is reduced by 33 as a benefit from the register. But overall, the register has up to now saved more than 11,000 revisions in 10 years. For the Swedish health care system, the quality registries have contributed to a significant cost reduction of in total US$140 million for THA alone.

The findings of Furnes et al. [20] regarding the economical impact of inferior implants in the Norwegian NAR give another example. They assessed the economic cost of using inferior implants and cements compared to a reference THA. The annual overall extra cost of using other implants than the reference THA was US$1.7 million for the first 3-5 years postoperatively. The register cost is estimated at $18 per case and decade in Norway [28].

14.11
International Registers

In recent years in Europe, several efforts have been started for both specific national registers and for a register covering all European countries. The European Federation of National Associations of Orthopaedics and Traumatology (EFORT) is one of the most influential organisations working on an European Arthroplasty Register (EAR). Based on the Scandinavian experience, avoidance of further implantation of inferior implant models in Europe must be the main goal. An international AR should be based on national registers which are available, function well and are organised by the respective national societies. However, EFORT is confronted with considerable problems as in most European countries no national AR exists and many countries still present the situation of uncontrolled implantation of a large number of inferior implants.

There must be a central unit, documenting all the data, but national ARs are responsible for the bias of their data. The control of the data security and correctness cannot be a task of an international EAR. But this separation may not be possible, because there are already plans in the European Union (EU) to legally specify an AR.

The structure of an EAR would have to be based upon a electronic information technology with common IT standards. A solution regarding this has not yetbeen found although corresponding technologies exist, even on modern web-based systems [56]. Keywords are web interface, digital image processing, optical mark readers, mobile barcode readers, computer-based web-server for patient and data privacy protection.

The advantages of an EAR are various. An international EAR provides the most effective and pragmatic approach for assessing the outcomes and quality of orthopaedic prostheses in Europe, as well as best practices, economic cost-effectiveness, incidences, prevalences and the requirednumbers of THA in Europe. An EAR would be an excellent resource for planning health services, aiding decision-making and carrying out health services research.

There is still further need to discuss the financing problems, the structure and control, and the leadership and organisation as well as the transparency and independence of such a central EAR. Decisions have not yet been taken. EFORT has the leading role in the realisation of this project.

References

1. Arcq M. Ectopic ossification: a complication after total hip replacement. Arch Orthop Unfallchir 1973 Nov 13;77(2):108–31
2. Bellamy N, Buchanan WW, Goldsmith CH, Campbell J, Stitt LW. Validation study of WOMAC: A health status instrument for measuring clinically important patient relevant outcomes to antirheumatic drug therapy in patients with osteoarthritis of the hip or knee. J Rheumatol 1988;15:1833–40
3. Bellamy N, Buchanan WW, Goldsmith CH, Campbell J, Stitt LW. WOMAC Osteoarthritis Index. A user's guide. University of Western Ontario, London, Ontario, Canada

4. Best AJ, Fender D, Harper WM, McCaskie AW, Oliver K, Gregg PJ. Current practice in primary total hip replacement: results from the National Hip Replacement Outcome Project. Ann R Coll Surg Engl 1998 Sep;80(5):350–5

5. Biedermann R, Krismer M, Stockl B, Mayrhofer P, Ornstein E, Franzen H. Accuracy of EBRA-FCA in the measurement of migration of femoral components of total hip replacement. Einzel–Bild–Rontgen–Analyse – femoral component analysis. J Bone Joint Surg Br 1999;81: 266–72

6. Biedermann R, Krismer M, Stöckl B, Mayrhofer P, Ornstein E, Franzén H. Accuracy of EBRA-FCA in the measurement of migration of femoral components of total hip replacement. J Bone Joint Surg Br 1999;81:266–72

7. Brooker AF, Bowerman JW, Robinson RA, Riley LH. Ectopic ossification following total hip replacement: incidence and a method of classification. J Bone Joint Surg Am 1973;55:1629

8. Bullinger M. Erfassung der gesundheitbezogenen Lebensqualität mit dem SF-36 Health Survey. Rehabilitation 1996;35:17–30

9. Callaghan JJ, Dysart SH, Savory CF, Hopkinson WJ. Assessing the results of hip replacement. A comparison of five different rating systems. J Bone Joint Surg Br 1990;72:1008–9

10. Decking J, Schuetz U, Decking R, Puhl W. The migration of femoral components after total hip replacement surgery: accuracy and precision of software-aided measurements. Skeletal Radiol 2003 Sep;32(9):521–5. Epub 2003 Jul 31

11. Dickob M, Bleher J, Puhl W. [Standardized analysis of acetabulum cup migration in hip endoprosthesis using digital image processing] Standardisierte Pfannenwanderungsanalyse in der Huftendoprothetik mittels digitaler Bildverarbeitung. Unfallchirurg 1994;97(2):92–7

12. Donabedian A. Explorations in quality assessment and monitoring. Voume I: The definition of quality and approaches to its assessments. Ann Arbor: Health Administration Pr, 1980

13. Effenberger H, Mechtler. Qualitätssicherung in der Hüftendoprothetik. In: Jerosch J, Effenberger H, Fuchs S (eds) Hüftendoprothetik. Stuttgart, NY: Thieme, pp. 68–78

14. Espehaug B, Havelin LI, Engesaeter LB, Vollset SE. The effect of hospital-type and operating volume on the survival of hip replacements. A review of 39,505 primary total hip replacements reported to the Norwegian Arthroplasty Register, 1988–1996. Acta Orthop Scand 1999 Feb;70(1):12–8

15. Fender D, Harper WM, Gregg PJ. Outcome of Charnley total hip replacement across a single health region in England: the results at five years from a regional hip register. J Bone Joint Surg Br 1999 Jul;81(4):577–81

16. Fender D, Harper WM, Gregg PJ. The Trent regional arthroplasty study. Experiences with a hip register. J Bone Joint Surg Br 2000 Sep;82(7):944–7

17. Fender D, van der Meulen JH, Gregg PJ. Relationship between outcome and annual surgical experience for the charnley total hip replacement. Results from a regional hip register. J Bone Joint Surg Br 2003 Mar;85(2):187–90

18. Frizelle DJ, Lewin RJ, Kaye G, Hargreaves C, Hasney K, Beaumont N, Moniz-Cook E. Cognitive-behavioural rehabilitation programme for patients with an implanted cardioverter defibrillator: A pilot study. Br J Health Psychol 2004 Sep;9(Pt 3):381–92

19. Furnes A, Havelin LI, Engesaeter LB, Lie SA. [Quality control of prosthetic replacements of knee, ankle, toe, shoulder, elbow and finger joints in Norway 1994. A report after the first year of registration of joint prostheses in the national registry]. Tidsskr Nor Laegeforen 1996 Jun 10;116(15):1777–81

20. Furnes A, Lie SA, Havelin LI, Engesaeter LB, Vollset SE. The economic impact of failures in total hip replacement surgery: 28,997 cases from the Norwegian Arthroplasty Register, 1987–1993. Acta Orthop Scand 1996 Apr;67(2):115–21

21. Furnes O, Lie SA, Espehaug B, Vollset SE, Engesaeter LB, Havelin LI. Hip disease and the prognosis of total hip replacements. A review of 53,698 primary total hip replacements

reported to the Norwegian Arthroplasty Register 1987–1999. J Bone Joint Surg Br 2001 May;83(4):579–86
22. Garellick G, Malchau H, Herberts P. Survival of hip replacements. A comparison of a randomized trial and a registry. Clin Orthop 2000 Jun;(375):157–67
23. Griss P. [Quality assurance in endoprosthetics]. Z Orthop Ihre Grenzgeb 1998 Mar-Apr;136(2): 95–6
24. Gruen TA, McNeice GM, Amstutz HC. "Modes of Failure" of cemented stem-type femoral components. A radiographic analysis of loosening. Clin Orthop 1979;141:17–27
25. Harris WH. Traumatic arthritis of the hip after dislocation and acetabular fractures: treatment by Mold arthroplasty. An end result study using a new method of results evaluation. J Bone Joint Surg AM 1969;51-A:737–55
26. Havelin LI, Engesaeter LB, Espehaug B, Furnes O, Lie SA, Vollset SE. The Norwegian Arthroplasty Register: 11 years and 73,000 arthroplasties. Acta Orthop Scand 2000 Aug;71(4):337–53
27. Havelin LI, Espehaug B, Vollset SE, Engesaeter LB, Langeland N. The Norwegian arthroplasty register. A survey of 17,444 hip replacements 1987–1990. Acta Orthop Scand 1993 Jun;64(3):245–51
28. Havelin LI. The Norwegian Joint Registry. Bull Hosp Jt Dis 1999;58(3):139–47
29. Hendrich C, Rader CP, Klein G, Oswald B, Kramer C. [Possibilities for interpreting digital migration analysis of cement-free PM total hip endoprostheses] Interpretationsmoglichkeiten der digitalen Wanderungsanalyse zementfreier PM-Hüfttotalendoprothesen. Z Orthop Grenzgeb 1997;135(4):285–91
30. Herberts P, Ahnfelt L, Malchau H, Stromberg C, Andersson GB. ulticenter clinical trials and their value in assessing total joint arthroplasty. Clin Orthop 1989 Dec;249:48–55
31. Herberts P, Malchau H. How outcome studies have changed total hip arthroplasty practices in Sweden. Clin Orthop 1997 Nov;344:44–60
32. Herberts P, Malchau H. Long-term registration has improved the quality of hip replacement: a review of the Swedish THA Register comparing 160,000 cases. Acta Orthop Scand 2000 Apr;71(2):111–21
33. Ingvarsson T, Hagglund G, Jonsson H Jr, Lohmander LS. Incidence of total hip replacement for primary osteoarthrosis in Iceland 1982–1996. Acta Orthop Scand 1999 Jun;70(3):229–33
34. Insall JN, Dorr LD, Scott R, Scott WN: Rationale of the knee society clinical rating system. Clin Orthop 1989;248:13–4
35. Johnston RC, Fitzgerald RH, Harris WH, Poss R, Müller ME, Sledge CB. Clinical and radiographic evaluation of total hip replacement. J. Bone Joint Surg 1990;72-A:161–8
36. Karrholm J, Borssen B, Lowenhielm G, Snorrason F. Does early micromotion of femoral stem prostheses matter? 4-7-year stereoradiographic follow-up of 84 cemented prostheses. J Bone Joint Surg Br 1994;76:912–7
37. Krismer M, Bauer R, Tschupik J, Mayrhofer P.: EBRA: a method to measure migration of acetabular components. J Biomech 1995;28(10):1225–36
38. Krismer M, Biedermann R, Stöckl B, Fischer M, Bauer R, Haid C. The prediction of failure of the stem in THA by measurement of early migration using EBRA–FCA. J Bone Joint Surg Br 1999;81:273–80
39. Krismer M, Tschupik JP, Bauer R, Mayrhofer P, Stöckl B, Fischer M, Biedermann R. Einzel–Bild–Röntgen–Analyse (EBRA) zur Messung der Migration von Hüftendoprothesen. Orthopäde 1997;26:229–36
40. Lang I, Willert HG. [Experiences with the German Endoprosthesis Register] Z Arztl Fortbild Qualitatssich 2001 Apr;95(3):203–8
41. Lucht U. The Danish Hip Arthroplasty Register. Acta Orthop Scand 2000 Oct;71(5):433–9
42. Malchau H, Herberts P, Eisler T, Garellick G, Soderman P. The Swedish Total Hip Replacement Register. J Bone Joint Surg Am 2002;84-A(suppl 2):2–20

43. Malchau H, Herberts P, Garellick G, Soderman P, Eisler T. Prognosis of total hip replacement: update of results and risk-ratio analysis for revision and re-revision from the Swedish National Hip Arthroplasty Register 1979-2000. Scientific Exhibition at the AAOS 2002, Dallas, USA
44. Malchau H, Herberts P, Söderman P, Oden A. Prognosis of total hip replacement: update and validation of results from the Swedish National Hip Arthroplasty Register 1979–1998. Scientific Exhibition at the AAOS 2000, Orlando, USA
45. Malchau H, Herberts P. Prognosis of total hip replacement: revision and re-revision rate in THA. A revision-risk study of 148,359 primary operations. Scientific Exhibition at the AAOS 1998, New Orleans, USA
46. Maloney WJ. National joint replacement registries: has the time come? J Bone Joint Surg Am 2001;83:1582–5
47. Merle d'Aubigné R, Cauchoix J, Ramadier JV. Evaluation chiffrée de la fonction de la hanche. Application à l'étude des résultats des opérations mobilisatrices de la hanche. Rev Chir Orthop 1949;35:541–8
48. Merle d'Aubigne R, Postel M. Functional results of hip arthroplasty with acryüc prosthesis. J Bone Joint Surg 1954;36-A:451–75
49. Merx H, Dreinhöfer K, Schräder P, Stürmer T, Puhl W, Günther KP, Brenner H. International variation in hip replacement. Ann Rheum Dis 2002;61:0–4
50. Müller R, Ghassem-Khanloo AA, Thümler P. Nachweis von minimalen Schaftwanderungen anhand von anterioposterioren Röntgenaufnahmen des Hüftgelenks. Orthopädische Praxis 1996;32(3):180–2
51. Müller R, Matuschek T, Thümler P. Digitale Röntgenbildbearbeitung zur Messung von Schaftwanderungen in der Hüftendoprothetik. Orthopädische Praxis 1996;32(3):177–9
52. Pitto RP, Lang I, Kienapfel H, Willert HG. The German Arthroplasty Register. Acta Orthop Scand Suppl 2002 Oct;73(305):30–3
53. Puolakka TJ, Pajamaki KJ, Halonen PJ, Pulkkinen PO, Paavolainen P, Nevalainen JK. The Finnish Arthroplasty Register: report of the hip register. Acta Orthop Scand 2001 Oct;72(5):433–41
54. Robertsson O, Knutson K, Lewold S, Lidgren L. The Swedish Knee Arthroplasty Register 1975-1997: an update with special emphasis on 41,223 knees operated on in 1988-1997. Acta Orthop Scand 2001 Oct;72(5):503–13
55. Robertsson O, Lewold S, Knutson K, Lidgren L. The Swedish Knee Arthroplasty Project. Acta Orthop Scand 2000 Feb;71(1):7–18
56. Röder C, El-Kerdi A, Eggli S, Aebi M. A centralized total joint replacement registry using web-based technologies. J Bone Joint Surg Am 2004;86:2077–9
57. Rothwell AG. Development of the New Zealand Joint Register. Bull Hosp Jt Dis 1999;58(3):148–60
58. Schuetz U, Decking J, Decking R, Puhl W. Assessment of femoral component migration in total hip arthroplasty. Digital measurements compared to RSA. Acta Orthop Belgica – accepted Dec 2004 (Issue 02/2004)
59. Soderman P, Malchau H, Herberts P, Johnell O. Are the findings in the Swedish National Total Hip Arthroplasty Register valid? A comparison between the Swedish National Total Hip Arthroplasty Register, the National Discharge Register, and the National Death Register. J Arthroplasty 2000 Oct;15(7):884–9
60. Soderman P, Malchau H, Herberts P, Zugner R, Regner H, Garellick G. Outcome after total hip arthroplasty: Part II. Disease-specific follow-up and the Swedish National Total Hip Arthroplasty Register. Acta Orthop Scand 2001 Apr;72(2):113–9
61. Soderman P, Malchau H, Herberts P. Outcome after total hip arthroplasty: Part I. General health evaluation in relation to definition of failure in the Swedish National Total Hip Arthoplasty register. Acta Orthop Scand 2000 Aug;71(4):354–9

62. Soderman P, Malchau H. Validity and reliability of Swedish WOMAC osteoarthritis index: a self-administered disease-specific questionnaire (WOMAC) versus generic instruments (SF-36 and NHP). Acta Orthop Scand 2000;71(1):39–46
63. Stucki G, Meier D, Stucki S, Michel BA, Tyndall AG, Dick W, Theiler R. Evaluation einer deutschen Version des WOMAC (Werstern Ontario und McMaster Universities) Arthroseindex. Zeitschrift für Rheumatologie 1996;Band 55, Heft 1:40–9
64. Walker PS, Mai SF, Cobb AG, Bentley G, Hua J. Prediction of clinical outcome of THA from migration measurements on standard radiographs. A study of cemented Charnley and Stanmore femoral stems. J Bone Joint Surg Br 1995;77:705–14

The Patient's View: Indicators of Subjective Health and Their Use in Outcome Assessment

15

T. Kohlmann

15.1
Introduction

The relevance of indicators reflecting the patient's view on outcomes of health care is increasingly recognized in clinical research and clinical practice. Explicit inclusion of the patient's personal experience of health and disease and of the risks and benefits of medical interventions has now become an accepted perspective in evaluative studies, medical decision making and health policy [11]. In particular, measures of *perceived health status* and *health-related quality of life* have been included in a growing number of studies published in the medical literature [13].

According to the context in which they are used, indicators of subjective health may be applied for different purposes. In *routine clinical practice*, they can be valuable tools for screening for potential problems, assessing patient preferences and monitoring change and outcomes in individual patients [14]. In *clinical trials*, the status of these measures depends on their role in the whole set of outcome criteria:

1. Indicators of subjective health may be used in clinical trials as *primary outcome parameters* in cases where, for example, subjectively experienced physical symptoms such as pain and fatigue or aspects of psychological well-being are the central focus of therapeutic efforts.
2. When relevant outcomes can be assessed by physician- and patient-reported measures, both approaches, objective and subjective measures, may provide valuable *complementary information*. Physical function and performance, ability to work and overall health status are examples of clinical outcomes which can be addressed from several methodological perspectives.
3. Self-reported measures may also be included in clinical trials as *additional criteria* for evaluating therapeutic benefit. Besides the main clinical outcomes, patient-reported

T. Kohlmann (✉)

Institute for Community Medicine, Walther-Rathenau-Str. 48, 17487 Greifswald, Germany

e-mail: thomas.kohlmann@uni-greifswald.de

K.E. Dreinhöfer et al. (eds.), *EUROHIP: Health Technology Assessment of Hip Arthroplasty in Europe*, DOI: 10.1007/978-3-540-74137-4_15, © 2009 EFORT

positive and negative side effects of treatment as well as patient satisfaction may be targets in a comprehensive evaluation of efficacy and safety.

During the last 20 years, a considerable number of validated instruments for measuring subjective health have been developed. These instruments for measuring the patient's perception of health can be divided into three broad categories: disease-specific, generic, and preference-based instruments. Disease-specific instruments are intended for use in a particular disease or set of similar conditions such as musculoskeletal, cardiovascular or respiratory diseases. As they address those dimensions of subjective health which are known to be important for a particular condition, it is commonly assumed that they should be more discriminative and responsive than generic instruments. Generic instruments, on the other hand, are developed to assess a wide range of different aspects of subjective health applicable to a variety of diseases. With their multi-dimensional approach, they cover health problems which may or may not be relevant for a specific condition. Their main advantage is that results obtained with these instruments can be directly compared across different patient groups and therapeutic interventions. Preference-based instruments are (mostly generic) single-index measures representing the "utility" of a given health state (on a scale from 0 to 1, for example). These instruments are useful for health economic studies and for calculating "quality-adjusted life-years" (QALYs). Some researchers are concerned about the possible insensitivity of preference-based measures because they aggregate multi-dimensional problems into a single index.

15.2
Patient-Reported Outcomes in Musculoskeletal Medicine

There is a fairly long tradition of measuring patient-reported aspects of health in musculoskeletal medicine [23]. Early developments of comprehensive, disease-specific instruments dating back to the 1970s demonstrated that major outcome criteria in rheumatology and orthopaedics can be reliably measured with patient-completed instruments. Meenan's Arthritis Impact Measurement Scales (AIMS) addressed several health problems including physical function (upper/lower extremities), psychological status (anxiety/depression), pain, and social activity [20]. This instrument was extensively tested and applied in studies of patients with rheumatic diseases. A revised and extended version was published 1992 (AIMS2 [21], cf. Table 15.1).

For use in patients with hip and knee osteoarthritis, Bellamy developed the Western Ontario and McMaster (WOMAC) Osteoarthritis Index (for a recent review, see [4]). This standardised questionnaire comprises 24 items that cover pain, stiffness and physical function. It is available in different formats and many languages, has been extensively validated and is now among the most commonly used self-reporting instruments for patients with hip or knee osteoarthritis [2]. Extended versions of the WOMAC instrument including additional dimensions and items were recently published [22, 24].

The Short-Form 36 (SF-36) and the Nottingham Health Profile (NHP) are examples of generic instruments for measuring health-related quality of life that have successfully been used in musculoskeletal medicine and other specialities [13]. Published studies comparing the SF-36 and NHP with specific measures like the WOMAC indicate that generic instruments may be slightly less sensitive to change [1, 7, 8]. However, there is increasing interest in generic

Table 15.1   Some examples of disease-specific, generic, and preference-based measures of subjective health

Instrument	No. of items	Scales
Disease-specific		
Arthritis Impact Measurement Scales 2 AIMS2 Meenan et al. [21]	66	Mobility level, walking and bending, hand and finger function, arm function, self-care, household tasks, social activities, support from family and friends, arthritis pain, work, level of tension, mood, satisfaction, arthritis impact
Western Ontario and McMaster Osteoarthritis Index WOMAC Bellamy [3]	24	Pain, stiffness, physical function
Generic		
Short-Form 36 Health Survey SF-36 Ware and Sherbourne [26]	36	Physical function, role-physical, bodily pain, general health, vitality, social function, role-emotional, mental health
Nottingham Health Profile NHP Hunt et al. [15]	38	Pain, energy, sleep, social isolation, emotional reactions, physical mobility
Preference-based		
EQ-5D EQ-5D EuroQol Group [9]	5	Overall index

instruments in musculoskeletal medicine because they enable direct comparisons between conditions and comparisons with published population norms. Furthermore, generic instruments may be more suitable for detecting unexpected side-effects or complications [5].

Preference-based instruments for measuring health-related quality of life are mainly applied in economic evaluation. The most widely used instrument in Europe is the EQ-5D questionnaire (or "EuroQol") comprising a "thermometer rating scale" and five items addressing, among others, problems with pain and discomfort, mobility, and anxiety and depression [6]. The EQ-5D has been included in several studies of patients with musculoskeletal conditions (rheumatoid arthritis, osteoarthritis) and has been shown to be sufficiently valid and responsive [5]. Yet, concern has been raised about its psychometric properties in specific patient samples [12, 27].

15.3
The Patient's View in Studies of Outcomes of Joint Replacement Surgery

Both disease-specific and generic patient-reported outcomes and measures of health-related quality of life have played a major role in evaluative studies of changes after hip or knee replacement surgery. It could be shown that many aspects of subjective health reflect significant and relevant improvement after joint replacement surgery. *Pain* and *functional limitations* are the main areas in which patients experience dramatic improvements [10]. As these positive patient-outcomes were also observed for older patients (75 years and over), researchers concluded that older age should not limit the access to arthroplasty [19].

Outcomes of hip replacement surgery have been compared with those of other *"high volume" elective procedures* using generic and specific measures of subjective health [28]. Changes in health-related quality of life as measured by the SF-36 were strongly positive after total hip replacement. On the whole, with up to 47% improvement, hip replacement resulted in greater changes than each of the other procedures included in the study (e.g. cholecystectomy, hysterectomy, lumbar diskectomy). Based on the WOMAC score, only 2% of the hip patients experienced a poor outcome 1 year after surgery.

The *dynamics of change* after joint replacement surgery have been addressed in a study of Bachmeier et al. [1]: For patients undergoing hip or knee joint replacement surgery, on average a 50% improvement in WOMAC scores 3 months after surgery was observed, followed by small but steady improvements during the following 9 months. Pain was in both groups the most responsive indicator. Improvements in WOMAC scores for pain, stiffness and physical function were more pronounced in the hip replacement group (Fig. 15.1).

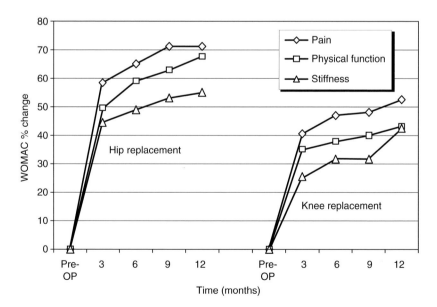

Fig. 15.1 Improvement after hip or knee joint replacement surgery shown as percent change in WOMAC scores from baseline (preoperation) to 3, 6, 9 and 12 months after surgery (Bachmeier et al. [1], calculated from entries in Figs. 1 and 2)

The SF-36 that was also included in the study of Bachmeier et al. was less responsive than the WOMAC scales but provided useful additional information. Hence, the authors concluded that application of both disease-specific and the generic instruments, especially in long-term studies, may give a more comprehensive account on the outcomes of hip and knee replacement surgery.

Mahon et al. [18] used the WOMAC in their study on the *impact of waiting* on outcomes after elective hip arthroplasty. While the length of waiting (≤6 months, >6 months) was not associated with postoperative WOMAC scores, patients waiting at least 6 months experienced clinically important increases in pain and reduced mobility before surgery, indicating a substantial impact of waiting on subjective health of patients with severe osteoarthritis of the hip.

In their study of patients drawn randomly from the hospital discharge register, Söderman et al. [25] demonstrated that the SF-36 and NHP can be successfully used for outcome evaluation after hip replacement. In addition, they compared survival rates of arthroplasties from the Swedish Hip Arthroplasty Register with rates of "clinical survival" in their patient sample. Clinical survival was defined by a combination of revision status and scores on the generic health measures. It could be shown that both indicators of failure, revision and subjective health, are useful end-points and can provide – if appropriately combined – valuable information about outcomes after hip arthroplasty.

15.4
Conclusion

It is widely accepted in many medical disciplines that evaluative studies should not only rely on traditional clinical outcomes but should also include outcome indicators representing the patient's perspective. This is of special importance in joint replacement surgery which is associated with clinically relevant, often dramatic, improvements in pain, physical functioning, mobility and other aspects of health status – all of these are genuine examples of patient-reported outcomes, of outcomes "that matter to patients". Examples of studies in which indicators of subjective health have been included demonstrate that focussing on the patient in outcome assessment can give a better insight into benefits of therapy than would be obtained by traditional clinical outcomes alone. If discrepancies between clinical and patient-reported outcomes are observed, this should not be considered a deficiency of either approach but another reason to include both perspectives for a comprehensive assessment [17].

Given the number and diversity of existing disease-specific, generic, and preference-based instruments, debate continues over the best choice of measures. Users may require guidance and recommendations for selecting appropriate instruments [16] but should also review results of comparative studies in samples of their target population. Ideally, a study would include all three types of instruments, but practical limitations will often result in a forced choice between them. While disease-specific measures may often provide more relevant information, generic and preference-based instruments are indispensable for comparisons across different conditions and economic evaluation, respectively.

References

1. Bachmeier CJM, March LM, Cross MJ, Lapsley HM, Tribe KL, Courtenay BG, Brooks PM. A comparison of outcomes in osteoarthritis patients undergoing total hip and knee replacement surgery. Osteoarthritis and Cartilage 2001; 9: 137–146
2. Beaton DE, Schemitsch E. Measures of health-related quality of life and physical function. Clinical Orthopaedics 2003; 413: 90–105
3. Bellamy N. Osteoarthritis – an evaluative index for clinical trials (MSc thesis). McMaster University, Hamilton, Ontario, Canada, 1982
4. Bellamy N. WOMAC: a 20-year experiential review of a patient-centered self-reported health status questionnaire. Journal of Rheumatology 2002; 29: 2573–2576
5. Brazier JE, Harper R, Munro J, Walters SJ, Snaith ML. Generic and condition-specific outcome measures for people with osteoarthritis of the knee. Rheumatology 1999; 38: 870–877
6. Brooks R, Rabin R, de Charro F (eds). The measurement and valuation of health status using EQ-5D: a European perspective. Dordrecht: Kluwer, 2003
7. Dawson J, Fitzpatrick R, Murray D, Carr A. Comparison of measures to assess outcomes in total hip replacement surgery. Quality in Health Care 1996; 5: 81–88
8. Escobar A, Quintana JM, Bilbao A, Azkárate J, Güenaga JI. Validation of the Spanish version of the WOMAC questionnaire for patients with hip or knee osteoarthritis. Clinical Rheumatology 2002; 21: 466–471
9. EuroQol Group. EuroQol – a new facility for the measurement of health-related quality of life. Health Policy 1990; 16: 199–208
10. Fitzgerald JD, Orav EJ, Lee TH, Marcantonio ER, Poss R, Goldman L, Mangione CM. Patient quality of life during the 12 months following joint replacement surgery. Arthritis and Rheumatism 2004; 51: 100–109
11. Fitzpatrick R, Davey C, Buxton MJ, Jones DR. Criteria for assessing patient based outcome measures for use in clinical trials. In: Stevens A, Abrams K, Brazier J, Fitzpatrick R, Lilford J (eds) The advanced handbook of methods in evidence based health care. London: Sage, 2001, pp. 181–194
12. Fransen M, Edmonds J. Reliability and validity of the EuroQol in patients with osteoarthritis of the knee. Rheumatology 1999; 38: 807–813
13. Garratt A, Schmidt L, Mackintosh A, Fitzpatrick R. Quality of life measurement: bibliographic study of patient assessed health outcome measures. BMJ 2002; 324: 1417–1419
14. Higginson IJ, Carr AJ. Using quality of life measures in the clinical setting. BMJ 2001; 322: 1297–1300
15. Hunt SM, McKenna SP, McEwen J, Backett EM, Williams J, Papp E. A quantitative approach to perceived health status: a validation study. Journal of Epidemiology and Community Health 1980; 34: 281–286
16. Jackowski D, Guyatt G. A guide to health measurement. Clinical Orthopaedics 2003; 413: 80–89
17. Lieberman JR, Dorey F, Shekelle P, Schumacher L, Kilgus DJ, Thomas BJ, Finerman GA. Outcome after total hip arthroplasty. Comparison of a traditional disease-specific and a quality of life measurement of outcome. Journal of Arthroplasty 1997; 12: 639–645
18. Mahon JL, Bourne RB, Rorabeck CH, Feeny DH, Stitt L, Webster-Bogaert S. Health-related quality of life and mobility of patients awaiting total hip arthroplasty: a prospective study. Canadian Medical Association Journal 2002; 167: 1115–1121
19. March LM, Cross MJ, Lapsley H, Brnabic AJM, Tribe KL, Machmeier CJM Courtenay BG, Brooks PM. Outcomes after hip or knee replacement surgery for osteoarthritis. Medical Journal of Australia 1999; 171: 235–238
20. Meenan RF, Gertman MP, Mason JH. Measuring health status in arthritis. The Arthritis Impact Measurement Scales. Arthritis and Rheumatism 1980; 23: 146–152

21. Meenan RF, Mason JH, Anderson JJ, Guccione AA, Kazis LE. AIMS2. The content and properties of a revised and expanded Arthritis Impact Measurement Scales Health Status Questionnaire. Arthritis and Rheumatism 1992; 35: 1–10
22. Nilsdotter AK, Lohmander LS, Klässbo M, Roos EM. Hip disability and osteoarthritis outcome score (HOOS) – validity and responsiveness in total hip replacement. BMC Musculoskeletal Disorders 2003; 4: 10 (www.biomedcentral.com/1471-2474/4/10)
23. Raspe H. Quality of life measurement in rheumatology. In Guggenmoos-Holzmann I, Bloomfield K, Brenner H, Flick U (eds) Quality of life and health. Oxford: Blackwell, 1995, pp. 97–106
24. Roos EM, Toksvig-Larsen S. Knee injury and osteoarthritis outcome score (KOOS) – validation and comparison to the WOMAC in total knee replacement. Health and Quality of Life Outcomes 2003; 1: 17 (www.hqlo.com/content/1/1/17)
25. Söderman P, Malchau H, Herberts P. Outcome after total hip arthroplasty. Part I. General health evaluation in relation to definition of failure in the Swedish National Total Hip Arthroplasty register. Acta Orthopaedica Scandinavica 2000; 71: 354–359
26. Ware JE, Sherbourne CD. The MOS 36-ltem Short-Form Health Survey (SF-36): I. Conceptual framework and item selection. Medical Care 1992; 30: 473–483
27. Wolfe F, Hawley DJ. Measurement of the quality of life in rheumatic disorders using the EuroQol. British Journal of Rheumatology 1997; 36: 786–793
28. Wright CJ, Chambers GK, Robens-Paradise Y. Evaluation of indications for and outcomes of elective surgery. Canadian Medical Association Journal 2002; 167: 461–466

The Perspectives when Assessing Function in Patients with Osteoarthritis

International Classification of Function, Disability and Health

16

K. Dreinhöfer, A. Cieza, and G. Stucki

At the launch of the Bone and Joint Decade, a WHO Scientific Group met on the burden of musculoskeletal conditions. Based on the results of that meeting, a recent WHO Technical Report suggests a number of health domains of importance in patients with osteoarthritis [1]. These recommendations are based on the health domains covered by available generic health status measures and a qualitative review of the literature. The domains include physical health, social health, mental health, and handicap/participation. In addition, this report mentions a number of sub-domains with different levels of importance, like pain, activities/roles, mobility, self care, eating, ambulation and sexuality.

The OMERACT (Outcome Measures in Rheumatology Clinical Trials) group has advised to always include the domains pain and physical function in Phase-III clinical trials and described stiffness as an important optional domain [2]. The OMERACT and the 5th WHO/ILAR Task Force (World Health Organisation/International League Against Rheumatism) [3, 4] recommended the use of condition-specific, health status measures including the Western Ontario and McMaster (WOMAC) Osteoarthritis Index [5] and the Lequesne-Algofunctional Index [6] to measure these domains in clinical research and practice. The current paradigm for the measurement of "function" or outcome assessment in osteoarthritis interventions is to use both, a condition-specific health status instrument and a generic health status instrument [7, 8]. These generic health status instruments (SF-36, EQ5D, NHP, MFA) assess domains relevant to patients with osteoarthritis, including dimensions of social function, emotional function, role function, pain and physical function. Recent publications have examined the sensitivity to change or responsiveness of the most widely used instruments in patients with osteoarthritis undergoing rehabilitation or surgical interventions [9–11]. Therefore, there is now a substantial body of knowledge about the performance of these instruments in patients undergoing osteoarthritis interventions.

However, the WOMAC index is a rather broad measure of physical functional disability, and encompasses some aspects relating to activities and participation, therefore overlapping with measures of generic health status. Since there is also an increasing interest in a

K. Dreinhöfer (✉)

Department of Orthopedics, Ulm University, Oberer Eselsberg 45, 89081 Ulm, Germany

e-mail: karsten.dreinhoefer@uni-ulm.de

K.E. Dreinhöfer et al. (eds.), *EUROHIP: Health Technology Assessment of Hip Arthroplasty in Europe*, DOI: 10.1007/978-3-540-74137-4_16, © 2009 EFORT

more differentiated measurement of condition-specific health status, it may be advantageous to differentiate a number of physical functional limitations in patients with osteoarthritis. Physical functional ability in patients with osteoarthritis can be differentiated in four factors: standing/walking, lying/sitting, bending, and climbing [12]. While a global measure such as the WOMAC may be ideal for epidemiological studies or registries, the use of the factor-based scales may be preferable when examining indications and outcomes for subsets of patients.

Condition-specific measures typically cover only selected aspects of the entire patient experience associated with osteoarthritis. These measures also vary in the concepts included [13, 14]. However, the patient experience of functioning and health goes beyond pain, stiffness and functional limitation with a focus on physical function. Also, in contrast to the OMERACT perspective, which focusses on functioning and health as an outcome of the disease process to be evaluated in phase-III trials, functioning and health is not merely an outcome, but the starting point for assessing functioning and health of patients.

Different from the approach of health-related quality of life, which has its focus on patient-reported outcomes, all aspects of the patient experience need to be covered, including activities and participation and also body functions and structures, as well as personal and environmental factors.

With the approval of the new international classification of functioning, disability and health (ICF) by the World Health Assembly in May 2001, a globally agreed-on etiologically neutral framework and a classification on the individual and population level exist. The ICF attempts to provide a coherent view of different perspectives of health from biological, individual and social perspectives. Patients' functioning is now seen as being associated with, and not merely a consequence of, a health condition [15]. Additionally, functioning and health are seen in relation to health conditions and also to personal and environmental factors. The ICF also overcomes the distinction between the healthy and the disabled, since functioning is seen along a continuum relevant to all people at some point in life. An individual's functioning in a specific domain is an interaction or complex relationship between the health condition and contextual factors (environmental and personal factors) (Fig. 16.1). There is a dynamic interaction among these entities, with intervention in one entity also having potential effects on the others.

The ICF consist of two parts: (1) *Functioning and Disability* with the two components *Body Functions and Structures* and *Activities and Participation* and (2) *Contextual Factors* with the components *Environmental Factors* and *Personal Factors*.

The components are interpreted by constructs. Body functions and structures are defined through changes in physiological systems or in anatomical structures. Activities and Participation are operationalised by the constructs *capacity* and *performance*. The basic construct of the component Environmental Factors is the facilitating or hindering impact of features of the physical, social and attitudinal world (*facilitators* or *barriers*). Personal Factors are not classified in the ICF because of the large social and cultural variance associated with them.

As a classification, the ICF provides the basis to describe the process of functioning and disability within health and health-related domains. The ICF *categories* represent the units of the classification and are designated by small letters: Body Functions (b), Body

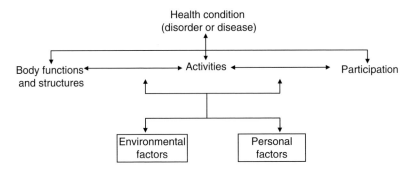

Fig. 16.1 Interaction between the components of the International Classification of Functioning, Disability and Health

Structures (s), Activities and Participation (d), and Environmental Factors (e). In the hierarchical code system, the letters are followed by a numeric code starting with the chapter number (one digit) followed by the second, third and fourth level digit. In each chapter there are therefore individual two-, three- or four-level categories.

A *health condition* is an umbrella term for disease, disorder, injury or trauma. It may also include other circumstances such as pregnancy, ageing, stress, congenital anomaly or genetic predisposition.

Functioning is an umbrella term for body functions, body structures, activities and participation and describes the positive aspects of the interaction between an individual with a health condition and the contextual factors of that individuum. *Disability* is an umbrella term for impairment, activity limitations and participation restrictions and denotes the negative aspects of the interaction between an individual and the contextual factors.

Body functions are the physiological functions of body systems including the brain. *Body structures* are the anatomical parts of the body such as organs, limbs and their components. *Impairment* is a loss or abnormality of physiological functioning (e.g. reduced range of motion, muscle weakness, pain and fatigue) or body structure (e.g. joints).

Activity is the execution of a task or action by an individual and represents the individual perspective of functioning, while *Participation* refers to the involvement of an individual in a life situation and represents the societal perspective of functioning. Difficulties of an individual in executing activities are denoted as *activity limitation* (e.g. limitations in mobility such as walking or climbing stairs), while problems experienced in life situations are referred to as *participation restriction* (e.g. restriction in community life, recreation and leisure).

Contextual factors represent the complete background of an individual's life and living situation. The *environmental factors* refer to all aspects of the physical, social and attitudinal environment in which people live and conduct their lives and, as such, have an impact on that person's functioning. *Personal factors* are contextual factors relating to the individual, but are not part of a health condition, i.e. age, gender, race, fitness, life-style and social status.

Risk factors can be described by personal factors (e.g. lifestyle, genetic kit, obesity) and by environmental factors (e.g. architectural barriers, living and working conditions). Risk

16

factors are not only associated with the onset, but can interact with the disabling process at each stage and affect the progression of the disease (e.g. treatment, rehabilitation, financial resources, expectations).

Different conditions are associated with different spectrums of abilities that are typically limited. Since the ICF consists of more then 1,400 categories, the development of disease-specific ICF Sets consisting of the most relevant domains is crucial for the usefulness and feasibility of this classification. Since the requirements to describe functioning in association with a condition are different for a multi-disciplinary comprehensive assessment of functioning, disability and health in patients with osteoarthritis and a clinical study or international registry, different ICF Core Sets are needed [15, 16].

The Comprehensive ICF Core Sets may guide the clinician when examining and taking the patient's history or deciding and evaluating interventions, while the Brief ICF Core Set should describe the prototypical spectrum of limitations of functioning and health in clinical studies. While the Comprehensive ICF Core Set should include all abilities that are typically limited in patients with a condition, the Brief ICF Core Set includes only the most relevant categories across cultures and countries to be practical in any situation or setting.

In an international approach led by the ICF Research Branch of the University of Munich and the CAS-Group at WHO and a number of cooperation partners and associated partners including the Bone and Joint Decade, a first version of a ICF Core Sets for osteoarthritis has been developed [17]. This involved a formal decision-making and consensus process integrating evidence gathered from preliminary studies including Delphi exercises [18], systematic reviews and an empiric data collection, using the ICF checklist [19].

In the consensus process' the varying spectrum of limitations in functioning in OA was addressed. In the early stage of the condition, the burden may be limited to minor and only sporadic symptoms. In the later stages, patients may experience a wide spectrum of functional impairments, activity limitations and participation restrictions in addition to now often more severe symptoms. Since ICF Core Sets need to capture the experience of all patients with OA independent of the stage, the joint involved or age, the participants included all categories that were considered relevant for patients with OA at some point. However, related co-morbidities and complications under consideration at all possible stages during the disease had to be excluded from the Core Sets. This should now allow the following of patients over time and the detecting of changes in the pattern of problems over time.

The Comprehensive ICF Core Set for the different components is presented in Tables 16.1a–16.1d. The ICF categories in bold represent the categories selected for the Brief ICF Core Set in the corresponding components. The total number of categories in the Comprehensive ICF Core Set is 55 (13 from the component body function, 6 body structure, 19 activities and participation and 17 environmental factors) and the Brief ICF Core Set includes a total number of 13 categories (3 each from the components body function, body structure, activities and participation, and 4 from environmental factors).

Limitations and restrictions in "activity and participation" as well as barriers in the "environmental factors" may indeed be most relevant to patients with OA. This is reflected by the fact that these component are represented by 19 and 17 categories, respectively, in the Comprehensive ICF Core Set, as compared with the 13 "body functions" considered relevant. Three of the five highest ranked categories in the Comprehensive ICF Core Set

Table 16.1a International Classification of Functioning, Disability and Health (ICF)-categories of the component "body functions" included in the Comprehensive ICF Core Set for osteoarthritis (from Dreinhöfer et al. [17])

ICF code	ICF category title
b130	Energy and drive functions
b134	Sleep functions
b152	Emotional functions
b280	Sensation of pain
b710	Mobility of joint functions
b715	Stability of joint functions
b720	Mobility of bone functions
b730	Muscle power functions
b735	Muscle tone functions
b740	Muscle endurance functions
b760	Control of voluntary movement functions
b770	Gait pattern functions
b780	Sensations related to muscles and movement functions

Table 16.1b International Classification of Functioning, Disability and Health (ICF)-categories of the component "body functions" included in the Comprehensive ICF Core Set for osteoarthritis (from Dreinhöfer et al. [17])

ICF code	ICF category title
s720	Structure of shoulder region
s730	Structure of upper extremity
s740	Structure of pelvic region
s750	Structure of lower extremity
s770	Additional musculoskeletal structures related to movement
S799	Structures related to movement, unspecified

belong to the domain "self-care". Beside the commonly reflected activities representing key issues for patients with OA, e.g. the domain "mobility", some categories that have not been addressed in most of the prior assessments like "recreation and leisure", "intimate relationships" and "remunerative employment" were included, since they are of great importance at least for a subgroup of patients [20].

One-third of the categories of the Comprehensive ICF Core Set belong to the component "environmental factors". "Products and technology" as well as "support and relationships", "attitudes" and "immediate family, friends, and societal attitudes" are highly important to patients with OA since they can serve as either a barrier or a facilitator. Cultural differences will have a serious impact on the applicability of some of the individual categories in different countries. The wide variety in total hip replacement rates, even in OECD countries [21], reflects the different "health services, systems and policies". However, as the developing world will account for a huge amount of the expected increase in OA prevalence globally, activities for improvement of OA-related health services in the individual countries are urgently required, including training and provision of "health professionals".

16

Table 16.1c International Classification of Functioning, Disability and Health (ICF)-categories of the component "activities and participation" included in the Comprehensive ICF Core Set for osteoarthritis (from Dreinhöfer et al. [17])

ICF code	ICF category title
d410	Changing basic body position
d415	Maintaining a body position
d430	Lifting and carrying objects
d440	Fine hand use
d445	Hand and arm use
d450	Walking
d455	Moving around
d470	Using transportation
d475	Driving
d510	Washing oneself
d530	Toileting
d540	Dressing
d620	Acquisition of goods and services
D640	Doing housework
D660	Assisting others
D770	Intimate relationships
D850	Remunerative employment
D910	Community life
D920	Recreation and leisure

Table 16.1d International Classification of Functioning, Disability and Health (ICF)-categories of the component "environmental factors" included in the Comprehensive ICF Core Set for osteoarthritis (from Dreinhöfer et al. [17])

ICF code	ICF category title
E110	Products or substances for personal consumption
E115	Products and technology for personal use in daily living
E120	Products and technology for personal indoor and outdoor mobility and transportation
E135	Products and technology for employment
E150	Design, construction and building products and technology of buildings for public use
E155	Design, construction and building products and technology of buildings for private use
E225	Climate
E310	Immediate family
E320	Friends
E340	Personal care providers and personal assistants
E355	Health professionals
E410	Individual attitudes of immediate family members
E450	Individual attitudes of health professionals
E460	Societal attitudes
E540	Transportation services, systems and policies
E575	General social support services, systems and policies
E580	Health services, systems and policies

If patients are scheduled for hip or knee replacement surgery, the disease is already in a late stage. At that time, nearly all patients suffer from pain and more than two-thirds have severe pain when walking. Many patients in this advanced stage report pain at night [22], one out of three arthritis patients suffers from sleep disturbances [23]. Half the patients have walked in the past 2 weeks less than one block, a quarter are only walking indoors. Every second patient needs assistance with walking and about one-third need assistance with housework or shopping [22]. In addition, depression is common in persons with OA [24]. Some patients may have a high preference regarding the importance of certain other problems, e.g. public transportation, unequal limb length, concerns about falling, the need to use walking aids and difficulty with recreational activities [25].

All these aspects are represented in the Comprehensive ICF Core Set, but only "sensation of pain" and "walking" are included in the Brief ICF Core Set. Some other main issues, e.g. concerns about falling and the loss of independence, are only represented indirectly by categories reflecting limitations in "moving around", "using transportation" and the "environmental factors". This clearly indicates the need to use the Comprehensive ICF Core Set in the assessment and follow-up of patients considering or undergoing joint replacement surgery. The breadth of ICF chapters contained in the Comprehensive ICF Core Set reflects the important and complex impairments, limitations and restrictions of activity and participation involved, as well as the numerous interactions with environmental factors.

These ICF Core Sets are preliminary and need to be tested extensively in the coming years in different countries, regions and cultures, in different subsets of patients with varying characteristics of patients and conditions, in the different health care settings and from the perspective of the different professions involved in the care of patients. As an example, OA of the hip and knee might severely affect the ability to participate in religious ceremonies in some parts of the world. However, the experts in the consensus process did not prioritise this category. The patient perspective has already been addressed in the empirical data collection of preliminary studies; however, the ICF Core Sets will need to undergo a close examination and possible modification by patient focus groups throughout the world.

When deciding on what to measure when studying osteoarthritis interventions, it is not ideal to simply decide on an instrument. Instead, it may be preferable to decide on the relevant domains first, based on the study endpoints, the population to be studied and the intervention, and only then to select the instrument to measure these domains.

The ICF allows for content comparison of different health status measures and provides information on which contents are covered by which health status measures [26]. Using linkage rules it is now possible to examine which condition-specific instruments and generic health status instruments best cover the domains considered to be relevant in the assessment of functioning, disability and health of patients with osteoarthritis [14]. The results of the linking process of the WOMAC and Lequesne-Algofunctional Index are shown in Table 16.2. The comparison of individual items of condition-specific and generic instruments using the ICF will also allow the detection of redundant items and may help to reduce the overlap of measurements in the future.

In conclusion, the ICF is an exciting landmark for the assessment of the impact of musculoskeletal conditions on the individual. The ICF is a comprehensive and adequate framework to assess the impact of health conditions on an individual level but also on a population level. While there will still be the need for a number of modifications and specific adaptations for specific requirements for the health status instruments, the ICF Core Sets provide

Table 16.2 Items of the WOMAC and the Lequesne-Algofunctional index and the corresponding ICF categories

WOMAC items	ICF-code	Lequesne items
Body functions		
3. Pain at night while in bed	b134 Sleep functions	1A–E: Pain or discomfort…
1.–5. Arthritis pain	b28016 Pain in joints	1B: Morning stiffness or regressive pain after rising
	b289 Sensation of pain, other specified and unspecified	1A–E: Pain or discomfort…
	b7603 Supportive functions of arm or leg	3D: Pain or discomfort while getting up from sitting without the help of arms
6. Stiffness after first wakening in the morning	b7800 Sensation of muscle stiffness or	1B: Morning stiffness or regressive pain after rising
7. Stiffness after sitting, lying or resting later in the day	b7808 Sensations related to muscles and movement functions, other specified	
Activities and participation		
10. Rising from sitting	d4100 Lying down	1B: Morning stiffness or regressive pain after rising
17. Rising from bed	d4101 Squatting	3C (hip): Squat or bend on the knees
12. Bending to floor	d4103 Sitting	1E (knee): Pain or discomfort while getting up from sitting without the help of arms
	d4105 Bending	3A (hip): Put on socks by bending forward
		3C (hip): Squat or bend on the knees
4. Pain sitting or lying	d4150 Maintaining a lying position	1A: Pain or discomfort during nocturnal bedrest
7. Stiffness after sitting, lying or resting later in the day		
19. Lying in bed		
4. Pain sitting or lying	d4153 Maintaining a sitting position	1E (hip): Pain or discomfort with prolonged sitting (2 h)
7. Stiffness after sitting, lying or resting later in the day		
21. Sitting		
5. Pain standing upright	d4154 Maintaining a standing position	1C: Pain or discomfort after standing for 30 min
11. Standing	d4400 Picking up	3B (hip): Pick up an object from the floor

Questionnaire item	ICF code	Description
1. Pain walking on a flat surface 13. Walking on flat surface	d4102 Transferring oneself while lying	1A: Pain or discomfort during nocturnal bedrest only on movement or in certain positions
	d4450 Walking	
	d4500 Walking short distances	2. Maximum distance walked (may walk with pain): – 1 km (in about 15 min) – From 500 to 900 m (in about 8–15 min) – From 300 to 500 m – From 100 to 300 m – Less than 100 m
	d4501 Walking long distances	2. Maximum distance walked (may walk with pain): Unlimited
2. Pain going up or down stairs 8. Descending stairs 9. Ascending stairs	d4502 Walking on different surfaces d4551 Climbing	3D (knee): Able to walk on uneven ground 3A (knee): climb up a 1 flight of stairs
14. Getting in/out of car 20. Getting in/out of bath 22. Getting on/off toilet 16. Putting on socks/stockings 18. Taking off socks/stockings 15. Going shopping 23. Heavy domestic duties 24. Light domestic duties	d4559 Moving around unspecified d498 Mobility, other specified d5101 Washing whole body d530 Toileting d5402 Putting on footwear d5403 Taking off footwear d6200 Shopping d699 Domestic life, unspecified	3B (knee): climb down 1 flight of stairs 1D: Pain or discomfort while ambulating 3D (hip): Can get into and out of a car
7. How severe is your stiffness after sitting, lying or resting later in the day?	d9208 Recreation and leisure, other specified	3A (hip): Put on socks by bending forward
Environmental factors		
	e1201 Assistive products and technology for personal indoor and outdoor mobility	2. Maximum distance walked (may walk with pain): with one walking stick or crutch

a stable and globally accepted reference. The ICF framework and applications such as the ICF Core Sets for osteoarthritis are likely to be used in clinical practice, outcomes and rehabilitation research, education, health statistics and regulation. Such generally-agreed-on lists of ICF categories can serve as ICF Core Sets to be rated in all patients included in a clinical study with OA or as Comprehensive ICF Core Set to guide multidisciplinary assessments in patients with OA. Large epidemiological studies or registries should therefore be aware of the ICF Core Set development and ensure that the most relevant domains covered by the ICF Core Sets are represented.

Acknowledgements The authors are grateful to the editors of *Osteoarthritis Cartilage* and the editor of the *Journal of Rehabilitation Medicine* for granting permission to use extracts and tables of previously published materials in this article.

References

1. WHO Scientific Group on the Burden of Musculoskeletal Conditions at the Start of the New Millennium. The burden of musculoskeletal conditions at the start of the new millennium. Geneva, 2003
2. Bellamy N, Kirwan J, Boers M, Brooks P, Strand V, Tugwell P, Altman R, Brandt K, Dougados M, Lequesne M. Recommendations for a core set of outcome measures for future phase III clinical trials in knee, hip, and hand osteoarthritis. Consensus development at OMERACT III. J Rheumatol 1997;24(4):799–802
3. Lequesne M. ILAR guidelines for testing slow acting drugs in osteoarthritis (SYSADOAs). Rev Esp Rheumatol 1993;20(suppl 1):220–1
4. Bellamy N. Outcome measurement in osteoarthritis clinical trials. J Rheumatol 1995;43 (suppl):49–51
5. Bellamy N, Buchanan WW, Goldsmith CH, Campbell J, Stitt LW. Validation study of WOMAC: a health status instrument for measuring clinically important patient relevant outcomes to antirheumatic drug therapy in patients with osteoarthritis of the hip or knee.J Rheumatol 1988;15(12):1833–40
6. Lequesne MG. The algofunctional indices for hip and knee osteoarthritis. J Rheumatol 1997;24(4):779–81
7. Dieppe PA. Recommended methodology for assessing the progression of osteoarthritis of the hip and knee joints. Osteoarthr Cartil 1995;3(2):73–7
8. Hawker G, Melfi C, Paul J, Green R, Bombardier C. Comparison of a generic (SF-36) and a disease specific (WOMAC) (Western Ontario and McMaster Universities Osteoarthritis Index) instrument in the measurement of outcomes after knee replacement surgery. J Rheumatol 1995;22(6):1193–6
9. Angst F, Aeschlimann A, Steiner W, Stucki G. Responsiveness of the WOMAC osteoarthritis index as compared with the SF-36 in patients with osteoarthritis of the legs undergoing a comprehensive rehabilitation intervention. Ann Rheum Dis 2001;60(9):834–40
10. Angst F, Aeschlimann A, Stucki G. Smallest detectable and minimal clinically important differences of rehabilitation intervention with their implications for required sample sizes using WOMAC and SF-36 quality of life measurement instruments in patients with osteoarthritis of the lower extremities. Arthritis Rheum 2001;45(4):384–91
11. Nilsdotter AK, Lohmander LS. Patient Relevant Outcomes after total hip replacement. A comparison between different surgical techniques. Health Qual Life Outcomes 2003;1(1):21–8

12. Ryser L, Wright BD, Aeschlimann A, Mariacher-Gehler S, Stucki G. A new look at the Western Ontario and McMaster Universities Osteoarthritis Index using Rasch analysis. Arthritis Care Res 1999;12(5):331–5
13. Prevalence of self-reported arthritis or chronic joint symptoms among adults - United States, 2001. MMWR Morb Mortal Wkly Rep 2002;51(42):948–50
14. Weigl M, Cieza A, Harder M, Geyh S, Amann E, Kostanjsek N, Stucki G. Linking osteoarthritis-specific health-status measures to the International Classification of Functioning, Disability, and Health (ICF). Osteoarthr Cartil 2003;11(7):519–23
15. Stucki G, Ewert T, Cieza A. Value and application of the ICF in rehabilitation medicine. Disabil Rehabil 2002;24(17):932–8
16. Stucki G, Cieza A, Ewert T, Kostanjsek N, Chatterji S, Ustun TB. Application of the International Classification of Functioning, Disability and Health (ICF) in clinical practice. Disabil Rehabil 2002;24(5):281–2
17. Dreinhöfer KE, Stucki G, Ewert T, Huber E, Ebenbichler G, Gutenbrunner C, Chatterji S, Cieza A. ICF core set for osteoarthritis. J Rehabil Med 2004;36(suppl 44):75–80
18. Weigl M, Cieza A, Andersen A, Kollerits B, Amann E, Füssl M, Stucki G. Identification of the most relevant ICF categories in patients with chronic health conditions: a Delphi exercise. J Rehabil Med 2004;44(suppl):12–21
19. Ewert T, Fuessl M, Cieza A, Andersen A, Chatterji S, Kostanjsek N, Stucki G. Indentification of the most common patient problems in patients with chronic conditions using the ICF check-list. J Rehabil Med 2004;44(suppl):22–9
20. Wright JG, Rudicel S, Feinstein AR. Ask patients what they want. Evaluation of individual complaints before total hip replacement. J Bone Joint Surg Br 1994;76(2):229–34
21. Merx H, Dreinhofer K, Schrader P, Sturmer T, Puhl W, Gunther KP, Brenner H. International variation in hip replacement rates. Ann Rheum Dis 2003;62(3):222–6
22. Holtzman J, Saleh K, Kane R. Gender differences in functional status and pain in a Medicare population undergoing elective total hip arthroplasty. Med Care 2002;40(6):461–70
23. Jordan JM, Bernard SL, Callahan LF, Kincade JE, Konrad TR, DeFriese GH. Self-reported arthritis-related disruptions in sleep and daily life and the use of medical, complementary, and self-care strategies for arthritis: the National Survey of Self-care and Aging. Arch Fam Med 2000;9(2):143–9
24. Frank R, Hagglund K. Mood disorders. Atlanta, GA: American College of Rheumatology, 1996
25. Wright JG, Young NL. The patient-specific index: asking patients what they want. J Bone Joint Surg Am 1997;79(7):974–83
26. Cieza A, Stucki G. Content comparison of health related quality of life (HRQOL) instruments based on the International Classification of Functioning, Disability and Health (ICF). Qual Life Res 2003;12(7):785

Conclusions: Where Do We Go from Here?

17

Karsten Dreinhöfer , Paul Dieppe, and Wolfhart Puhl

The work presented in this book is ongoing. The investigators who have contributed chapters remain research active in the field and continue to make important observations that are aiding improved understanding of the provision of hip joint replacement within developed countries. But, like much good science, their work has led to as many new questions as answers.

Those who have to pay for joint replacement and manage their provision in hospitals want answers, not new questions. They want to be able to plan provision and predict costs and outcomes. If we are to help them with their problems we need to understand the "patient pathway" – we need to know how and why some people with a bad hip get a joint replacement while others do not, we need to understand why some get a better outcome than others, and we need to be able to define best practice.

There are several things that the work presented here, along with the current literature available, tells us that we do know about hip replacement. Here are some of those "facts":

- Hip replacement is a highly effective and cost-effective intervention for advanced osteoarthritis that reduces pain and disability markedly in the majority of those who have the intervention.
- A minority of those operated on do not gain greatly from the procedure.
- There is no consensus about the indications for hip joint replacement.
- There are no known effective alternatives for people with severe hip disease.
- Rates of hip joint replacement continue to rise in most developed countries, and this trend is likely to continue in view of increasing longevity in those countries.
- Demand for primary hip replacement in the developing world, and of revision surgery in the developed world, are also increasing rapidly.
- Large, mostly unexplained, variations in provision rates exist between and within countries.
- There are also huge variations in the peri-operative care provided, types of prosthesis used, costs of the procedure and outcomes seen between different countries and in different provider units in the same country.

K. Dreinhöfer (✉)
Department of Orthopedics, Ulm University, Oberer Eselsberg 45, 89081 Ulm, Germany
e-mail: karsten.dreinhoefer@uni-ulm.de

K.E. Dreinhöfer et al. (eds.), *EUROHIP: Health Technology Assessment*
of Hip Arthroplasty in Europe, DOI: 10.1007/978-3-540-74137-4_17, © 2009 EFORT

17

But these "facts" point out the huge gaps in our knowledge and understanding. For example, we do not know when in the course of arthritis it is best to operate – should we do the hip replacement early on in the development of osteoarthritis, or should we wait until the individual is severely disabled? The answer to this question could have huge implications for health service delivery, as if we were to conclude that patients should be operated on much earlier in the evolution of their disease, the need for services would increase even more rapidly than we predict at present. Another key area of ignorance is our lack of understanding of variations in practice and provision. We do not know why rates of hip replacement vary so greatly in different parts of the developed world, nor do we know why the ways in which care is provided at and around the time of surgery vary so greatly, or how much difference those variations make to the outcomes. There is also the vexing problem that some of our patients who seem appropriate cases for surgery do not gain much improvement in pain or disability in spite of this major, irreversible and expensive operation. That shows that we still have problems with indications and patient selection. An allied problem is that it remains unclear how we should best assess outcomes. Finally, there is the question of cost-containment, on which we remain inappropriately ignorant.

The "Eurohip" project is trying to contribute answers to some of those questions. Others working within the auspices of the Bone and Joint Decade are doing similar work in other countries.

However, an ongoing general problem with research in fields such as ours is that much of it is too far removed from the problems of patients or of health care purchasers and managers. We now know a lot more about the technical problems and biological issues surrounding hip joint replacement than we do about service provision. Our hope is that this book and the work of both the "Eurohip" consortium and the "Bone and Joint Decade" will help the search for answers to the very practical questions.

Participants of the EUROHIP Project

Country		Participating Department	
Austria	Innsbruck	Department of Orthopaedics Innsbruck University Anichstraße 35 6020 Innsbruck	Prim. Univ. Prof. Dr. Martin Krismer Dr. med. Bernd Stoeckl
	Vienna	2. Orthopädische Abteilung Orthopedic Spital Wien–Speising Speisinger Straße 109 1130 Wien	Prim. Univ. Prof. Dr. Karl Knahr Oswald Pinggera
Finland	Helsinki	Orton Orthopaedic Hospital The Invalid Foundation Tenholantielo 10, 00280 Helsinki	Dr. Pekka Ylinen
France	Paris	Groupe Hospitalier Cochin Service du Chirurgie Orthopedique 27, rue du Faubourg, Saint-Jacques 75679 Paris Cedex 14	Prof. Moussa Hamadouche
	Lyon	Clinique Emilie de Vialar 116, Rue Antoine Charial 69003 Lyon	Dr. Jacques Henri Caton
	Longjumeau	Clinique de L'yvette 43, Route de Corbeil 91160 Longjumeau	Dr. Christian Delaunay
	Toulouse	Centre Hospitalier Ranguell Avenue du Pr J. Poulhes 31059 Toulouse	Prof. Philippe Chiron
Germany	Ulm	Department of Orthopaedics University of Ulm Oberer Eselsberg 45 89081 Ulm	Prof. Dr. med. Wolfhart Puhl Dr. med. Karsten Dreinhöfer Dr. med. Markus Flören Dr. Dagmar Gröber-Grätz, MPH
	Dresden	Department of Orthopaedics Universitätsklinikum Carl Gustav-Carus Fetscherstr. 74 01307 Dresden	Prof. Dr. med. Klaus-Peter Günther Dr. med. Stefan Fickert
	Heidelberg	Orthopädische Universitätsklinik Heidelberg Schlierbacher Landstraße 200a 69118 Heidelberg	Prof. Dr. med. Volker Ewerbeck Dr. med. Peter Aldinger Dr. med. Dominik Parsch

Country		Participating Department	
	Hamburg	Endo-Klinik Holstenstr. 2 22767 Hamburg	Prof. Dr. med. Joachim Löhr Dr. med. Alexander Katzer Dr. med. Dietrich Klüber
	Mannheim	Orthopädische Universitätsklinik Mannheim Theodor-Kutzer-Ufer 1-3 68167 Mannheim	Prof. Dr. med. Hanns-Peter Scharf Dr. med. Peter Schräder Dr. med. Sabine Schmitt
	Magdeburg	Orthopädische Universitätsklinik der Otto von Guericke Universität Magdeburg Leipziger Str. 44 39120 Magdeburg	Prof. Dr. med. Neumann Dr. med. Ingmar Meinecke Dr. med. Olof Bittner
Hungary	Szeged	Department of Orthopaedics University of Szeged Semmelweis-Str. 6 6725 Szeged	Dr. med. Kellermann Dr. med. Ildiko Fistzer
Iceland	Akureyri	General Hospital University Hospital 600 Akureyri	Dr. Thorvaldur Ingvarsson
Italy	Torino	Clinica Ortopedica I Universita degli Studi di Torino Dipartimento di Traumatologia, Ortopedia e Medicina del Lavoro Via Zuretti 29 10126 Torino	Prof. Paolo Gallinaro Dr. Alessandro Masse
Poland	Warsaw	Department of Orthopaedics Medical University of Warsaw 4 Lindley st. 02-005 Warsaw	Prof. Andrzej Górecki Maciek Ambroziak
Spain	Madrid	Orthopaedic Department Hospital La Paz Paseo de la Castellana 261 28046 Madrid	Prof. Eduardo Garcia-Cimbrelo
	Helsingborg	Department of Orthopedics Helsingborg Hospital 25187 Helsingborg	Anna Nilsdotter, MD, PhD Urban Benger, MD
	Karlsham	Department of Orthopaedics Blekingesjukhuset 37480 Karlshamm	Christian Hellerfelt, MD Christer Olson, MD
Sweden	Lund	Department of Orthopaedics Surgery University of Lund 22185 Lund	Prof. Stefan Lohmander, MD, PhD
	Malmö	Faculty of Medicine Department of Orthopaedics Malmö University Hospital 205 02 Malmö	Prof. Olof Johnell, MD, PhD

Country		Participating Department	
Switzerland	Aarau	Kantonspital Aarau Orthopädische Klinik Buchserstraße 5000 Aarau	Dr. Joerg Huber Ivan Broger
	Zurich	Rheuma- und Rehabilitationsklinik Stadtspital Triemli Birmesdorferstr. 497 8063 Zürich	Priv.-Doz. Dr. med. Robert Theiler Dr. med, Kurt Uehlinger Dr. med. Angela Hett
UK	Bristol	Medical Research Council Health Services Research Collaboration Department of Social Medicine University of Bristol BS8 2PS	Paul Dieppe Victoria Cavendish Susan Williams
	Bristol	Winford Unit Avon Orthopaedic Center Southmead Hospital Bristol BS10 5NB	Prof. Ian Learmonth
	Dundee	University Department of Orthopaedics & Trauma Surgery Ninewells Hospital and Medical School Dundee DD1 9SY	Prof. David Rowley
USA	Boston	Div. of Pharmacoepidemiology and Pharmacoeconomics Brigham and Women's Hospital Harvard Medical School Boston MA 02115	MPH

Printing: Krips bv, Meppel, The Netherlands
Binding: Stürtz, Würzburg, Germany